Cardiovascular Emergencies

Guest Editors

J. STEPHEN BOHAN, MD
JOSHUA M. KOSOWSKY, MD

EMERGENCY MEDICINE CLINICS OF NORTH AMERICA

www.emed.theclinics.com

Consulting Editor
AMAL MATTU, MD

November 2011 • Volume 29 • Number 4

SAUNDERS an imprint of ELSEVIER, Inc.

W.B. SAUNDERS COMPANY

A Division of Elsevier Inc.

1600 John F. Kennedy Boulevard • Suite 1800 • Philadelphia, Pennsylvania 19103-2899

http://www.theclinics.com

EMERGENCY MEDICINE CLINICS OF NORTH AMERICA Volume 29, Number 4
November 2011 ISSN 0733-8627, ISBN-13: 978-1-4557-1095-9

Editor: Patrick Manley

Emergency Medicine Clinics of North America (ISSN 0733-8627) is published quarterly by Elsevier Inc., 360 Park Avenue South, New York, NY, 10010-1710. Months of issue are February, May, August, and November. Business and Editorial Offices: 1600 John F. Kennedy Boulevard, Suite 1800, Philadelphia, PA 19103-2899. Customer Service Office: 6277 Sea Harbor Drive, Orlando, FL 32887-4800. Periodicals postage paid at New York, NY, and additional mailing offices. Subscription prices are $142.00 per year (US students), $281.00 per year (US individuals), $478.00 per year (US institutions), $201.00 per year (international students), $404.00 per year (international individuals), $576.00 per year (international institutions), $201.00 per year (Canadian students), $347.00 per year (Canadian individuals), and $576.00 per year (Canadian institutions). International air speed delivery is included in all *Clinics'* subscription prices. All prices are subject to change without notice. **POSTMASTER:** Send address changes to *Emergency Medicine Clinics of North America*, Elsevier Periodicals Customer Service, 11830 Westline Industrial Drive, St. Louis, MO 63146. Customer Service (orders, claims, online, change of address): Elsevier Periodicals Customer Service, 11830 Westline Industrial Drive, St. Louis, MO 63146. Tel: 1-800-654-2452 (U.S. and Canada); 314-453-7041 (outside U.S. and Canada). Fax: 314-453-5170. E-mail: journalscustomerservice-usa@elsevier.com (for print support); journalsonline support-usa@elsevier.com (for online support).

Reprints. For copies of 100 or more of articles in this publication, please contact the Commercial Reprints Department, Elsevier Inc., 360 Park Avenue South, New York, NY 10010-1710. Tel.: 212-633-3812; Fax: 212-462-1935; E-mail: reprints@elsevier.com.

Emergency Medicine Clinics of North America is covered in *MEDLINE/PubMed (Index Medicus), Current Contents/Clinical Medicine, EMBASE/Excerpta Medica, BIOSIS, SciSearch, CINAHL, ISI/BIOMED,* and *Research Alert.*

Printed and bound by CPI Group (UK) Ltd, Croydon, CR0 4YY

Transferred to Digital Print 2011

Contributors

CONSULTING EDITOR

AMAL MATTU, MD, FAAEM, FACEP
Program Director, Emergency Medicine Residency; Professor, Department of Emergency Medicine, University of Maryland School of Medicine, Baltimore, Maryland

GUEST EDITORS

J. STEPHEN BOHAN, MD
Executive Vice Chair, Emergency Medicine; Associate Physician, Brigham and Women's Hospital; Assistant Professor of Medicine, Harvard Medical School, Boston, Massachusetts

JOSHUA M. KOSOWSKY, MD
Department of Emergency Medicine, Brigham and Women's Hospital, Boston, Massachusetts

AUTHORS

JOHN P. BENNER, BA, NREMT-P
Charlottesville-Albemarle Rescue Squad, Charlottesville; Virginia College of Osteopathic Medicine, Blacksburg, Virginia

MATTHEW J. BIVENS, MD
Resident, Harvard-Affiliated Emergency Medicine Residency, Department of Emergency Medicine, Beth Israel Deaconess Medical Center, Boston, Massachusetts

LAURA J. BONTEMPO, MD
Assistant Professor, Department of Emergency Medicine, Yale University, New Haven, Connecticut

WILLIAM J. BRADY, MD
Department of Emergency Medicine, University of Virginia School of Medicine; Charlottesville-Albemarle Rescue Squad; Albemarle County Fire Rescue, Charlottesville, Virginia

RICHARD S. CHEN, MD, MBA
Resident, Harvard-Affiliated Emergency Medicine Residency, Department of Emergency Medicine, Beth Israel Deaconess Medical Center, Boston, Massachusetts

KATHERINE DOLBEC, MD
Department of Emergency Medicine, Maine Medical Center, Portland, Maine

ERIC GORALNICK, MD
Instructor, Department of Emergency Medicine, Brigham and Women's Hospital and Harvard Medical School, Boston, Massachusetts

SHAMAI A. GROSSMAN, MD, MS
Assistant Professor of Medicine, Harvard Medical School; Director, Clinical Decision Unit and Cardiac Emergency Center; Department of Emergency Medicine, Beth Israel Deaconess Medical Center, Boston, Massachusetts

JOSHUA M. KOSOWSKY, MD
Department of Emergency Medicine, Brigham and Women's Hospital, Boston, Massachusetts

NATHAN W. MICK, MD, FACEP
Director, Pediatric Emergency Medicine; Assistant Professor, Department of Emergency Medicine, Maine Medical Center, Portland, Maine

SARAH MORRIS, MD
Department of Emergency Medicine, University of Virginia School of Medicine, Charlottesville, Virginia

ALLAN R. MOTTRAM, MD
Assistant Professor, Division of Emergency Medicine, Department of Medicine, University of Wisconsin School of Medicine and Public Health, Madison, Wisconsin

PETER S. PANG, MD, FAAEM, FACEP
Associate Professor, Department of Emergency Medicine; Associate Professor, Center for Cardiovascular Innovation, Department of Medicine, Northwestern University Feinberg School of Medicine, Chicago, Illinois

DALE P. QUIRKE, MD
Attending Physician, Bay Area Emergency Physicians, Clearwater, Florida

JAMES E. SVENSON, MD
Associate Professor, Division of Emergency Medicine, Department of Medicine, University of Wisconsin School of Medicine and Public Health, Madison, Wisconsin

ANTHONY J. WEEKES, MD
Clinical Associate Professor of Emergency Medicine, Department of Emergency Medicine, University of North Carolina, Chapel Hill; Director, Emergency Ultrasound Fellowship, Department of Emergency Medicine, Carolinas Medical Center, Charlotte, North Carolina

KATHLEEN WITTELS, MD
Clinical Instructor in Medicine (Emergency Medicine), Harvard Medical School; Attending Physician, Department of Emergency Medicine, Brigham and Women's Hospital, Boston, Massachusetts

MAAME YAA A.B. YIADOM, MD, MPH
Physician, Department of Emergency Medicine, Cooper University Hospital; Researcher, The Cooper Heart Institute; Clinical Instructor, Robert Wood Johnson Medical School, Camden, New Jersey

Contents

therapies with a 3-phased approach for out-of-hospital resuscitation from ventricular fibrillation and pulseless ventricular tachycardia. Although this model is not a new concept, it is largely based on the 2010 AHA Guidelines, enhancing the philosophy of the "CAB" concept (Chest compressions/Airway management/Breathing rescue).

Patients who present to the ED with chest pain (or its equivalent) but have no electrocardiographic changes or elevation in cardiac biomarkers after an appropriate interval can be considered low risk for acute coronary syndrome. Combined with a low demographic risk for coronary artery disease (eg, using Framingham criteria), such patients can be said to be "low risk" for a subsequent coronary event. Whether there is a role for further risk stratification with provocative testing and/or coronary imaging before discharge remains open to debate.

Patients with cardiac rhythm disturbances may present in a variety of conditions. Patients may be unstable, requiring immediate interventions, or stable, allowing for a more deliberated approach. Rapid assessment of patient stability, underlying rhythm, and determination of appropriate interventions guides timely therapy. This article discusses the differential diagnosis and treatment of adult patients presenting with primary bradydysrhythmias and tachydysrhythmias, with the exception of atrial fibrillation and atrial flutter, covered elsewhere in this issue. A concise approach to diagnosis and determination of appropriate therapy is presented.

Atrial fibrillation (AF) results from the chaotic depolarization of atrial tissue and is the most common dysrhythmia diagnosed in United States (US) emergency departments. AF affects greater than 1% of the general population, with a peak prevalence of 10% in those greater than 80 years of age. By 2050, it is estimated that nearly 16 million US patients will suffer from AF. AF has significant health effects, and places a considerable economic burden on the health care system. This article discusses recommendations that are derived from a combination of existing guidelines, additional evidence, and consensus.

Emergency echocardiography refers to the use of cardiac ultrasound to address critical and time-sensitive clinical questions during the initial evaluation and treatment of the patient. The information obtained can be pivotal to a physician's clinical decision making and can guide further diagnostic or therapeutic interventions. This article provides an evidence-based discussion of the common uses of emergency transthoracic echocardiography, as well as its benefits and limitations in the current practice of emergency medicine.

Kathleen Wittels

Aortic emergencies present a diagnostic and treatment challenge for emergency physicians. Both acute aortic dissection and abdominal aortic aneurysms can be difficult to recognize, and a missed or delayed diagnosis may be fatal. A high clinical suspicion and rapid patient evaluation are important. Although many patients ultimately require surgical intervention, early and aggressive attention to hemodynamic stability by the emergency physician can provide a window to definitive treatment.

Richard S. Chen, Matthew J. Bivens, and Shamai A. Grossman

A popular saying holds that if one can hear a heart murmur in the middle of a loud and busy emergency department, then by definition the murmur is significant. Whether or not this is actually true, it does capture the frustration emergency physicians feel when trying to diagnose or manage valvular pathologic conditions with familiar yet limited tools. This article focuses on the valve-related issues the emergency physician will face, from the trauma patient with a mechanical valve who may need his or her anticoagulation reversed to the febrile patient with a new murmur.

Katherine Dolbec and Nathan W. Mick

Pediatric congenital heart disease comprises a wide spectrum of structural and electrical defects. These lesions present in a limited number of ways. An infant presenting with profound shock, cyanosis, or evidence of congestive heart failure should raise the suspicion of congenital heart disease. Although most congenital lesions are diagnosed in utero, the emergency physician must be aware of these cardinal presentations because many patients present in the postnatal period around the time that the ductus arteriosus closes. Aggressive management of cardiopulmonary instability combined with empiric use of prostaglandin E1 and early pediatric cardiology consultation is essential for positive outcomes.

GOAL STATEMENT

The goal of *Emergency Medicine Clinics of North America* is to keep practicing physicians up to date with current clinical practice in emergency medicine by providing timely articles reviewing the state of the art in patient care.

ACCREDITATION

The *Emergency Medical Clinics of North America* is planned and implemented in accordance with the Essential Areas and Policies of the Accreditation Council for Continuing Medical Education (ACCME) through the joint sponsorship of the University of Virginia School of Medicine and Elsevier. The University of Virginia School of Medicine is accredited by the ACCME to provide continuing medical education for physicians.

The University of Virginia School of Medicine designates this enduring material activity for a maximum of 15 *AMA PRA Category 1 Credit*(s)™ for each issue, 60 credits per year. Physicians should claim only the credit commensurate with the extent of their participation in the activity.

The American Medical Association has determined that physicians not licensed in the US who participate in this CME enduring material activity are eligible for a maximum of 15 *AMA PRA Category 1 Credit*(s)™ for each issue, 60 credits per year.

The Emergency Medicine Clinics of North America CME program is approved by the American College of Emergency Physicians for 60 hours of ACEP Category I Credit per year.

Credit can be earned by reading the text material, taking the CME examination online at http://www.theclinics.com/home/cme, and completing the evaluation. After taking the test, you will be required to review any and all incorrect answers. Following completion of the test and evaluation, your credit will be awarded and you may print your certificate.

FACULTY DISCLOSURE/CONFLICT OF INTEREST

The University of Virginia School of Medicine, as an ACCME accredited provider, endorses and strives to comply with the Accreditation Council for Continuing Medical Education (ACCME) Standards of Commercial Support, Commonwealth of Virginia statutes, University of Virginia policies and procedures, and associated federal and private regulations and guidelines on the need for disclosure and monitoring of proprietary and financial interests that may affect the scientific integrity and balance of content delivered in continuing medical education activities under our auspices.

The University of Virginia School of Medicine requires that all CME activities accredited through this institution be developed independently and be scientifically rigorous, balanced and objective in the presentation/discussion of its content, theories and practices.

All authors/editors participating in an accredited CME activity are expected to disclose to the readers relevant financial relationships with commercial entities occurring within the past 12 months (such as grants or research support, employee, consultant, stock holder, member of speakers bureau, etc.). The University of Virginia School of Medicine will employ appropriate mechanisms to resolve potential conflicts of interest to maintain the standards of fair and balanced education to the reader. Questions about specific strategies can be directed to the Office of Continuing Medical Education, University of Virginia School of Medicine, Charlottesville, Virginia.

The faculty and staff of the University of Virginia Office of Continuing Medical Education have no financial affiliations to disclose.

The authors/editors listed below have identified no professional or financial affiliations for themselves or their spouse/partner:
John P. Benner, BA, NREMT-P; Matthew J. Bivens, MD; Stephen Bohan, MD (Guest Editor); Laura J. Bontempo, MD; William J. Brady, MD; Richard S. Chen, MD, MBA; Katherine Dolbec, MD; Eric Goralnick, MD; Shamai A. Grossman, MD, MS; Joshua M. Kosowsky, MD (Guest Editor); Patrick Manley, (Acquisitions Editor); Amal Mattu, MD (Consulting Editor); Nathan W. Mick, MD; Sarah Morris, MD; Allan R. Mottram, MD; Dale P. Quirke, MD; James E. Svenson, MD; Anthony J. Weekes, MD; Kathleen Wittels, MD; Bill Woods, MD (Test Author); and Maame Yaa A.B. Yiadom, MD, MPH.

The authors/editors listed below identified the following professional or financial affiliations for themselves or their spouse/partner:
Peter S. Pang, MD is a consultant for Bayer, Medtronic, Novartis, Otsuka, SigmaTau, Trevena; receives honoraria from J & J, the Medicines Company, and Corthera; and receives research support from Abbott.

Disclosure of Discussion of Non-FDA Approved Uses for Pharmaceutical Products and/or Medical Devices.
The University of Virginia School of Medicine, as an ACCME provider, requires that all faculty presenters identify and disclose any off-label uses for pharmaceutical and medical device products. The University of Virginia School of Medicine recommends that each physician fully review all the available data on new products or procedures prior to clinical use.

TO ENROLL

To enroll in the Emergency Medicine Clinics of North America Continuing Medical Education program, call customer service at 1-800-654-2452 or visit us online at www.theclinics.com/home/cme. The CME program is available to subscribers for an additional fee of $190.00.

Foreword

Cardiovascular Emergencies

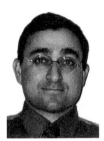

Amal Mattu, MD
Consulting Editor

Ask any emergency physician to list the most common chief complaints among emergency department (ED) patients and chest pain is certain to show up as a top complaint. Ask those same emergency physicians to list the most deadly conditions in the ED and you're likely to see acute myocardial infarction, dysrhythmias, and perhaps an assortment of other cardiac conditions. Next, ask risk managers and malpractice lawyers for their "top 5" list of causes of malpractice in emergency medicine and, once again, you're certain to see cardiac conditions on that list. In short, cardiac conditions are common, deadly, and high risk from a medicolegal standpoint. A sound knowledge of emergency cardiology is an absolute prerequisite to the successful practice of emergency medicine.

Further highlighting the importance of emergency cardiology is the fact that the largest portion of the emergency medicine core curriculum and the largest section of nearly every textbook in emergency medicine is the section on cardiology. Emergency cardiac conditions are the most common lecture topics at major conferences and usually the most highly attended lectures. Emergency cardiology research studies are often the most commonly published and read articles in the major journals. All of us in the emergency medicine community struggle to achieve competency in this area of emergency medicine by wading through the many publications and attending many lectures on these topics, and we hope that our efforts will be effective.

Rarely, however, we have the good fortune to see a publication that brings all of the latest advances in emergency cardiology in a single source. Drs Steve Bohan and Joshua Kosowsky have brought us such a resource. As guest editors, they've assembled an excellent set of authors who have reviewed the current literature and written a series of concise updates to guide our practice through numerous high-risk cardiac topics. The reader will quickly gain knowledge of the most recent updates pertaining to diagnosis and management of patients with acute coronary syndromes (ACS). The recent ACS Guidelines of the American College of Cardiology and American Heart Association (AHA) are reviewed in detail. The authors also review other important

Emerg Med Clin N Am 29 (2011) xi–xii
doi:10.1016/j.emc.2011.09.020
0733-8627/11/$ – see front matter © 2011 Elsevier Inc. All rights reserved.

guidelines including those pertaining to acute heart failure and atrial fibrillation. Other acute dysrhythmias and cardiac arrest are discussed, and in doing so the most recent AHA resuscitation guidelines ("Advanced Cardiac Life Support") are addressed. Valvular heart disease and congenital heart disease, both of which are topics that emergency physicians often have less familiarity, are also addressed in detail. Finally, an article is devoted to emergency bedside echocardiography, a skill that has not been a traditional component of most emergency physicians' repertoire but is certainly gaining importance in our practice.

To state that this issue of *Emergency Medicine Clinics* is a valuable addition to the library of emergency physicians is an understatement. This issue should be considered must-reading for all emergency health care providers, including trainees. Knowledge and practice of the concepts that are discussed in the following pages are certain to save lives and prevent lawsuits. The guest editors and authors are to be commended for providing this outstanding resource that will educate us all on a common, deadly, and medicolegally high-risk topic.

Amal Mattu, MD
Department of Emergency Medicine
University of Maryland School of Medicine
110 S. Paca Street, 6th Floor, Suite 200
Baltimore, MD 21201, USA

E-mail address:
amattu@smail.umaryland.edu

Preface

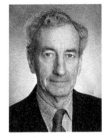 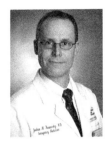

J. Stephen Bohan, MD   Joshua M. Kosowsky, MD
Guest Editors

There was a time in the long distant past when a cardiac emergency meant it was time to call a cardiologist. Then along came "time is muscle" and with it a stunning recognition that there was a different group of physicians who worked under the mantra of "Any Patient, Any Time" and who could commonly attend to the patient in five minutes or less. The stage was set and it became apparent that the care of acute cardiovascular conditions was squarely within the purview of Emergency Medicine.

Cardiovascular emergencies are notable for their sudden onset and often require quick thinking and quick action in response. It was with this in mind that we prepared this volume: to enhance real-time clinical decision-making with practical information, evidence-based where evidence is available and expert-consensus-based where it is not.

Our evidence base grows by the day and is much more clinically oriented than in the past, dealing not only with new diagnostic tools (novel biomarkers, bedside ultrasound) and treatments (new anti-thrombotic agents, non invasive ventilation) but also with processes (how best to achieve rapid door-to-balloon times, which chest-pain patients can go home at the end of the Emergency Department visit).

Our authors are masters of their respective topics, having been immersed in the literature on it long before we tapped them to share it with you the reader. Their exposition is clear, purposeful, uncluttered, and, blessedly, short. In something between 15 and 30 minutes you can also become a master of a topic with up-to-date information and a wealth of clinical pearls. See a patient, read the article, and never look back—until the next edition at least.

J. Stephen Bohan, MD

Joshua M. Kosowsky, MD
Department of Emergency Medicine
Brigham and Women's Hospital
10 Vining Street
Boston, MA 02115, USA

E-mail addresses:
JBOHAN@PARTNERS.ORG (J.S. Bohan)
jmkosowsky@partners.org (J.M. Kosowsky)

Emerg Med Clin N Am 29 (2011) xiii
doi:10.1016/j.emc.2011.10.002
0733-8627/11/$ – see front matter © 2011 Elsevier Inc. All rights reserved.

Acute Heart Failure Syndromes: Initial Management

Peter S. Pang, MD[a,b],*

KEYWORDS

• Acute heart failure • Initial management • Clinical profiles

Patients with acute heart failure syndromes (AHFS) are defined as those who present with heart failure (HF) signs and symptoms in need of urgent or emergent therapy.[1] More than 1 million hospitalizations for AHFS occur every year, at a cost of more than $20 billion dollars.[2] HF is the costliest and most common cause of readmission for Medicare beneficiaries.[3] Post-discharge mortality and re-hospitalization affects approximately 45% of discharged patients within 90 days.[4] Attempts to improve these post-discharge event rates with novel therapies have largely failed.[5]

Robust evidence to guide clinicians on initial therapeutic management is lacking; there are no class I, level A (best evidence) recommendations regarding the use of any therapy for initial AHFS management.[6] Despite the lack of robust evidence, smaller studies and expert opinion suggest a consensus approach to early management. Readers are referred to other textbooks for a more detailed explanation of epidemiology and pathophysiology. This article focuses on initial emergency department (ED) therapeutic management.

More than 6 million persons in the United States have a diagnosis of HF with more than 550,000 new diagnoses each year.[7] Of the 1 million annual AHFS admissions, approximately 80% initially present to the ED.[8] The aging of the population, combined with more patients living longer after myocardial infarction, will likely lead to an increased public health burden of HF.[5]

Approximately half of AHFS admissions are female, and approximately half have a relatively preserved ejection fraction (EF >40%).[9,10] The heterogeneity of the patient population is perhaps its most unifying characteristic; patients with AHFS have multiple comorbid cardiac and noncardiac conditions.

Despite significant reductions in cardiovascular morbidity and mortality over the last 10 years, post-discharge death and re-hospitalization from AHFS remains high,

a Department of Emergency Medicine, Northwestern University Feinberg School of Medicine, Chicago, IL, USA
b Center for Cardiovascular Innovation, Department of Medicine, Northwestern University Feinberg School of Medicine, Chicago, IL, USA
* Department of Emergency Medicine, 211 E Ontario St, Suite 200, Chicago, IL 60641.
E-mail address: ppang@northwestern.edu

Emerg Med Clin N Am 29 (2011) 675–688
doi:10.1016/j.emc.2011.08.004
0733-8627/11/$ – see front matter © 2011 Elsevier Inc. All rights reserved.

affecting ~45% of the discharged population within 90 days.[4] Inpatient mortality remains relatively low, ranging from 4% to 9%.[1,8,9,11] Attempts to improve these outcomes with novel therapies have failed, with no new therapy demonstrating any safe reduction in mortality and/or rehospitalization.[12–17]

At present, there are no class I, level A therapeutic guideline recommendations for AHFS.[6] Present-day therapies, such as oxygen, noninvasive ventilation, intravenous (IV) loop diuretics, morphine, and nitrates are the same therapies used 40 years ago.[18] Small studies as well as retrospective analyses suggest that the most commonly used therapy, IV loop diuretics, are associated with harm, including mortality, worsening renal function, and neurohormonal activation.[19] Yet although no conclusive data exist, decades of use support both its safety and effectiveness at improving signs and symptoms.

Whether supportive evidence for traditional therapies will be forthcoming (eg, randomized controlled trials) is unknown. Given this important contextual caveat, that robust evidence is lacking, a framework for ED management of AHFS is presented.

INITIAL APPROACH TO PATIENTS WITH AHFS

Prompt recognition and treatment of any life-threatening illness is the first priority for any patient presenting with signs and symptoms of AHFS. This article assumes that, in the management of AHFS, there is no other precipitant or cause that is of greater treatment priority and that AHFS is a manifestation of that precipitant. For example, a patient who presents with ST-segment elevation myocardial infarction (STEMI) and AHFS, treatment of STEMI is the first priority.

DIAGNOSIS

An initial approach to ED management of AHFS is shown in **Table 1**.[20] Because patients present with signs and symptoms rather than a diagnosis, ensuring that the patient has AHFS versus another diagnosis is a critical step, but is not always easy, because signs and symptoms of AHFS are also seen in other disease states. The most common symptom reported by patients is dyspnea or breathlessness.[21] The most specific physical examination findings are an S3 and jugular venous distention (JVD).[22] A chest radiograph without evidence of volume overload (eg, vascular engorgement or interstitial edema) does not rule out acute HF.[20] Patients with chronic heart failure adapt to a volume-overloaded state; thus radiographic features may be absent.[23,24]

In the last 10 years, natriuretic peptides (NP) have established both their diagnostic and prognostic roles.[25] When an HF diagnosis is in doubt, a brain natriuretic peptide (BNP) level less than 100 pg/mL largely rules out AHFS, whereas a level greater than 400 pg/mL rules in AHFS. However, these are guides and neither very high nor very low levels absolutely rule AHFS in or out. N-terminal probrain natriuretic peptide (NT-proBNP) levels have the same role, although threshold levels differ based on age.[25] From a prognostic standpoint, higher NP levels are independently associated with worse outcomes.[25] Use of NPs has been associated with shorter length of stay, decreased time to treatment, and even improved outcomes in AHFS; however, for some of these findings, further prospective studies are needed.[25–28]

DETERMINE THE CLINICAL PROFILE AND BEGIN THERAPY

Dividing patients based on their presenting characteristics is recommended, given the heterogeneity of the patient population. However, prospective evidence to support

Table 1
Initial approach to ED management of AHFS

	Initial Management for AHFS[a]
1. Treat immediate life-threatening conditions/stabilize patient	Life-saving measures may precede or parallel diagnostic evaluation (ie, unstable arrhythmia, flash pulmonary edema, STEMI)
2. Establish the diagnosis	Based on medical history, signs (JVD, S[3], edema), symptoms (dyspnea), biomarkers (eg, BNP) and CXR
3. Determine clinical profile and begin initial treatment	Key components include HR, BP, JVP, presence of pulmonary congestion, ECG, CXR, renal function, troponin, BNP, pulse oximetry, history of CAD
4. Determine and manage the cause or precipitant	Such as ischemia, hypertension arrhythmias, acute valvular disorders, worsening renal function, uncontrolled diabetes, and/or infectious causes is critical to ensure maximal benefits from HF management
5. Alleviate symptoms (eg, dyspnea)	Usually a diuretic with or without other vasoactive agents. Morphine may also be used for pulmonary edema[b]
6. Protect/preserve myocardium and renal function	Avoid hypotension or increase in HR, particularly in patients with CAD. Use of inotropes should be restricted to those with low-output state (low BP with organ hypoperfusion)
7. Make disposition	Most are admitted to telemetry, with a small number discharged home. Robust evidence to support risk stratification and disposition identifying the low-risk patient for safe discharge with close outpatient follow-up is lacking

Abbreviations: BNP, brain natriuretic peptide; CAD, coronary artery disease; CXR, chest radiograph; ECG, electrocardiogram; HR, heart rate; JVD, jugular venous distention; JVP, jugular venous pressure.
[a] These steps usually occur in parallel, not in series.
[b] Retrospective data suggest that morphine is associated with worse outcomes.
From Gheorghiade M, Pang PS. Acute heart failure syndromes. J Am Coll Cardiol 2009;53(7): 564; with permission.

this approach is minimal and is based largely on smaller studies and expert consensus opinion.[29] Multiple approaches have been proposed[1,20,30]; central to all such proposals is the overlap between groups. The approach recommended here divides patients based on initial systolic blood pressure, an important prognostic marker.[4,29]

The presented framework (**Fig. 1**) broadly divides patients with AHFS into 3 categories: (1) hypertensive (systolic blood pressure [SBP] >140 mm Hg) (**Fig. 2**), (2) normotensive (SBP 90–140 mm Hg) (**Fig. 3**), (3) hypotensive (SBP<90 mm Hg) (**Fig. 4**), with a distinct initial approach for each profile. Because the clinical approach is described in each figure, it is not repeated in the text.

THERAPEUTIC CONSIDERATIONS
Noninvasive Ventilation

In acute pulmonary edema, studies have shown the benefit of noninvasive ventilation (NIV) to reduce intubation rates, through improved oxygenation and decreased work

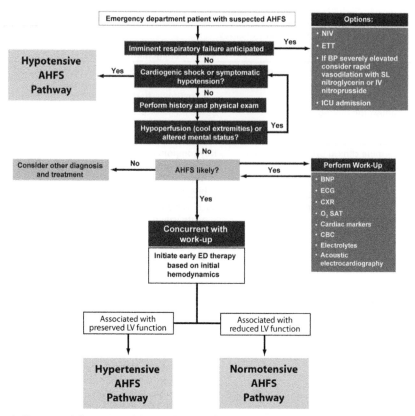

Fig. 1. Framework for categorizing patients with AHFS. BP, blood pressure; CXR, chest radiograph; ECG, electrocardiogram; ICU, intensive care unit; LV, left ventricular; O₂SAT, oxygen saturation; CBC, complete blood count; ED, emergency department; ETT, endotracheal tube; NIV, non-invasive ventilation; SL, sub-lingual.

of breathing.[31,32] because the studies to support these benefits have been small, the 3CPO trial (Cardiogenic Pulmonary Edema, n = 1069) was conducted, which concluded that there were no differences between NIV and standard oxygen therapy in terms of death or intubation rates within 7 days.[31]

Despite this evidence from a well-designed clinical trial, which is arguably the strongest evidence for any AHFS therapy to date, most emergency physicians continue to anecdotally report the benefits of NIV. These benefits are especially noted in the absence of any significant safety concerns with short-term use, assuming appropriate patients are chosen. Thus, despite the 3CPO trial results, this author recommends NIV in patients who present with acute cardiogenic pulmonary edema. Specifically, 10 to 15 cm H₂O is recommended as a starting point with continuous positive airway pressure. Patients often improve rapidly, or, if the intervention is without benefit, it may be easily removed.

IV Loop Diuretics

Dosing recommendations for initial IV diuretic therapy vary. The American Heart Association (AHA)/American College of Cardiology (ACC) recommend a dose at least equal to the oral dose for those on chronic oral diuretic therapy.[6] It is not clear whether this

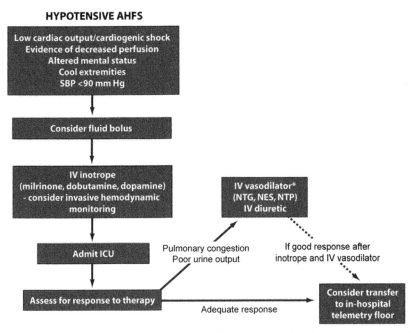

Fig. 2. Hypotensive AHFS pathway. NES, nesiritide; NTG, nitroglycerin; NTP, nitroprusside.

should equal the total oral dose upfront or be divided. The European Society of Cardiology (ESC) recommends 20 to 100 mg of IV furosemide, depending on the severity of presentation.[30] Similar to other therapies commonly used in AHFS, the evidence on which to base definitive guidelines for dosing are lacking because of the absence of large, well-powered trials showing its efficacy and safety. The recently published DOSE-AHF trial showed no differences between continuous versus bolus diuretic

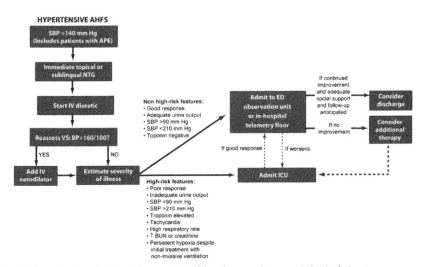

Fig. 3. Hypertensive AHFS pathway. BUN, blood urea nitrogen; VS, vital signs.

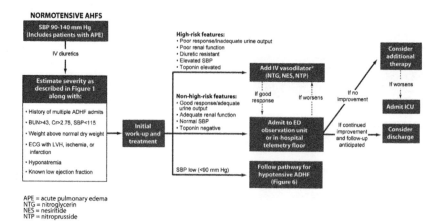

APE = acute pulmonary edema
NTG = nitroglycerin
NES = nesiritide
NTP = nitroprusside

Fig. 4. Normotensive AHFS pathway. Cr, creatinine; ICU, intensive care unit; LVH, left ventricle hypertrophy.

dosing. However, their high-dose arm, defined as 2.5 times the oral dose divided over a 24-hour period, showed significantly greater urine output as well as greater dyspnea improvement and weight loss, albeit with a transient worsening of renal function. No differences in mortality or rehospitalization were seen at 60 days. The inclusion criteria allowed for enrollment up to 24 hours after presentation; whether enrolling patients in the ED would have led to different conclusions is unknown.

The DOSE-AHF trial suggests that higher doses may be given safely. Thus, this author recommends, as a general rule, that twice the total chronic oral dose be administered in divided doses over a 24-h period, and started in the ED. For example, if a patient is on 80 mg of oral furosemide twice a day, and your institution primarily uses twice-daily dosing, 160 mg IV is recommended as the initial starting dose. If dosing 3 times a day is more common, then 80 mg IV should be given. Reassessment of the patient, both clinically as well as in terms of urine output, is critical.

Vasodilators

Large registry data suggest that most patients are primarily treated with IV loop diuretics.[33] However, both the hypertensive and normotensive management algorithms highlight the important role of vasodilator therapy. (Unless otherwise specified, vasodilators refers to nitroglycerin.) Previous research suggests both the safety and efficacy of vasodilators at improving signs and symptoms, and potentially outcomes.[34–36] If IV nitroglycerin is not readily available, sublingual or nitroglycerin sprays should be used in appropriate patients. A general guide based on ESC guidelines for where to start dosing and titration is shown in **Table 2**. Given the rapid onset and short half-life of IV nitroglycerin, rapid uptitration is possible with adjustment based on clinical improvement. Fears of taking an intensive care unit (ICU) bed are unfounded; depending on local circumstances, IV nitroglycerin can often be used to stabilize the patient initially. After diuresis has begun, topical nitropaste can then be applied and the IV nitroglycerin weaned.

Early Use of Angiotensin-converting Enzyme Inhibitors

Use of sublingual angiotensin-converting enzyme inhibitors (ACEI) or IV ACEI has been given a class C recommendation or expert consensus approval by the American

Table 2
Use of vasodilators. Indications and dosing of IV vasodilators in acute HF

Vasodilator	Indication	Dosing	Main Side Effects	Other
Nitroglycerine	Pulmonary congestion/ edema BP≥90 mm Hg	Start 10–20 µg/min increase to 200 µg/min	Hypotension, headache	Tolerance on continuous use
Isosorbide dinitrate	Pulmonary congestion/ edema BP≥90 mm Hg	Start with 1 mg/h, increase to 10 mg/h	Hypotension, headache	Tolerance on continuous use
Nitroprusside	Hypertensive HF congestion/ edema BP≥90 mm Hg	Start with 0.3 µg/kg/min and increase to 5 µg/kg/min	Hypotension, isocyanate toxicity	Light sensitive
Nesiritide	Pulmonary congestion/ edema BP≥90 mm Hg	Bolus 2 µg/kg + infusion 0.015– 0.03 µg/kg/min	Hypotension	—

Reproduced from Dickstein K, Cohen-Solal A, Filippatos G, et al. ESC Guidelines for the diagnosis and treatment of acute and chronic heart failure 2008: the Task Force for the Diagnosis and Treatment of Acute and Chronic Heart Failure 2008 of the European Society of Cardiology. Developed in collaboration with the Heart Failure Association of the ESC (HFA) and endorsed by the European Society of Intensive Care Medicine (ESICM). Eur Heart J 2008;29(19):2341; with permission.

College of Emergency Physicians (ACEP) clinical policy committee.[37] However, the ESC clearly recommends against the early use of ACEI to stabilize AHFS.[30] The differences lie in which studies are used as the basis for the recommendations. Small studies of early ACEI suggest its benefit at reducing SBP and alleviating symptoms.[37] However, well-powered studies that definitively show efficacy at reducing signs and symptoms and, more importantly, outcomes have yet to be performed. There is a paucity of safety data, with retrospective analysis suggesting potential harm in certain populations.[38] The idea that early neurohormonal blockade with ACEI is beneficial is often postulated, but unproved. Given the existence of other effective therapies, namely nitrates, with a long-standing tradition of empirical use as well as higher levels of evidence to support their use as supported by guidelines, use of ACEI is not recommended by this author until adequately powered studies are performed. The primary rationale lies in the potential risk for harm coupled with the availability of other agents.

Nesiritide

Use of nesiritide decreased considerably after retrospective analyses suggested potential safety concerns; namely worsening renal function and mortality.[39–41] Largely because of these concerns, the largest trial conducted to date in AHFS, the ASCEND-HF trial (Acute Study of Clinical Effectiveness of Nesiritide in Decompensated Heart Failure) with more than 7000 patients, was conducted with results presented at the end of 2010.[17] Briefly, the safety of nesiritide was well established, but the co-primary efficacy end points (mortality reduction or rehospitalization within 30 days and dyspnea improvement at 6 and 24 hours) were not reached. The improvement in dyspnea seen in previous studies was not duplicated.[34]

Table 3
Past modeling studies with reported outcomes and variables found to be significant risk indicators

Author, Year	N	Subject Type	Study Type	Outcome	Significant Variables
Filippatos, 2007	302	I	R	60-d death/readmission	BUN>40 mg/dL
Gheorghiade et al, 2007	48,612	I	R	In-hospital and 30-d mortality	Na^{2+}<135 mmol/L
Formiga, 2007	414	I	R	In-hospital mortality	Barthel index, creatinine, edema
Diercks, 2006[a]	499	E	P	LOS<24 h, 30-d events	SBP, troponin I
Rohde, 2006	779	I	R	In-hospital mortality	SBP<124 mm Hg, Cr>1.4 mg/dL, BUN>37 mg/dL, Na<136 mmol/L
Gheorghiade et al, 2006	48,612	I	R	In-hospital and 30-d mortality	SBP<120
Barsheshet, 2006	1122	I	R	In-hospital mortality	Age, glucose, female sex, creatinine, low SBP, NYHA class III/IV
Burkhardt, 2005	385	I	R	Observation unit discharge	BUN
Auble, 2005[a]	33,533	I	R	Inpatient complications and mortality	Na^{2+}, SBP, white blood cell count, pH, creatinine
Fonarow, 2005	65,275	I	R	Inpatient mortality	BUN, creatinine, SBP
Klein, 2005	949	I	R	Days hospitalized in 2 mo	Na^{2+}
Felker, 2004	949	I	R	60-d mortality/readmission	Age, SBP, BUN, Na^{2+}, Hgb, no. of past admissions, class IV symptoms
Lee, 2003	4031	I	R	30-d and 1-y mortality	Age, SBP, RR, BUN, Na^{2+}
Harjai, 2001	434	I	R	30-d readmission	Sex; COPD; prior admissions

Study	N	Setting	Method	Outcome	Markers
Butler, 1998	120	I	R	Inpatient complications	O_2 saturation; creatinine; pulmonary edema
Villacorta, 1998	57	I	R	Inpatient/6-mo death	Na^{2+}; sex
Chin, 1997	257	I	R, S	60-d readmission/death	Marital status; comorbidity index; admit SBP; No ST-T changes
Chin, 1996	435	I	R	Inpatient complications	Initial SBP; RR; Na^{2+}; ST-T changes
Selker, 1994	401	I	PA, R	Inpatient mortality	Age; SBP; T-wave flattening; HR
Brophy, 1993	153	E	P	LOS and 6-mo mortality	Left atrial size; cardiac ischemia; diuresis
Esdaile, 1992	191	I	PA, R	Inpatient mortality	Age; chest pain; cardiac ischemia; valvular disease; arrhythmia; new onset; poor response
Katz, 1988	216	E	R	2-d complications	4-h diuresis; history of pulmonary edema; T-wave abnormalities; JVD
Plotnick, 1982	55	I	PA, R	Inpatient and 1-y mortality	Admit SBP; dyspnea; peak CPK

Complications include mortality.

Abbreviations: COPD, chronic obstructive pulmonary disease; CPK, creatine phosphokinase; E, emergency department patients; Hgb, hemoglobin; I, inpatients; LOS, length of stay; NYHA, New York Health Association; PA, patient assessment; R, retrospective chart review; S, survey.

[a] Identified markers of low risk.

Reproduced from Collins SP, Storrow AB. Acute heart failure risk stratification: can we define low risk? Heart Fail Clin 2009;5(1):79, vii; with permission.

At present, consistent with guideline recommendations, nesiritide may be used as a vasodilator in AHFS. An additional advantage compared with nitroglycerin is that an ICU setting is not required. However, this author recommends its use as a second-line agent when nitrates are either not working or insufficient during the ED phase of management. The argument regarding nitrate tolerance does not usually apply in the ED setting.

Morphine

Similar to other traditional therapies, the evidence regarding morphine use in AHFS is limited. Its primary benefit lies in its vasodilatory properties as well as anxiolysis; however, retrospective analysis suggests morphine is associated with worse outcomes.[42–44] Guidelines are again split regarding this issue, with the Society for Chest Pain Centers recommending against the early use of morphine, whereas the ESC guidelines allow for early use, albeit with caution for respiratory depression, and recognition of the limited prospective studies on which to base this recommendation.[30,44]

This author limits use of morphine to the perinoninvasive ventilation setting, because the tight fitting mask may provoke some anxiety.

DETERMINE AND TREAT THE PRECIPITANT

Diagnosis and management of the precipitant for decompensation occurs in parallel with treatment. Common precipitants are seen in **Fig. 3**. Although medication and dietary indiscretion remain important considerations, treatable or reversible causes of decompensation are critical to identify and treat.

SPECIAL CONSIDERATIONS
Hypotensive Profile

Patients presenting with low SBP are rare. The temptation to immediately raise the blood pressure should be tempered by careful consideration of the overall clinical picture combined with investigation of the patient's baseline state. Patients with end-stage or advanced HF may have reduced systolic function to such a degree that low SBP may be normal or baseline.

Inotropic agents are reserved for those patients with cardiogenic shock or evidence of hypoperfusion. Both the ESC and the AHA/ACC guidelines mention that inotropes may lead to increased risk of both short-term and longer-term adverse events.[6,30] However, both guidelines also recommend their use for patients in need of such supportive therapy. Given the infrequent nature of such presentations, emergent consultation with cardiology is also recommended.

Atrial Fibrillation and HF

The management of patients with atrial fibrillation (AF) and rapid ventricular response (RVR) and HF present a unique challenge. Although controlling the rate is the common reaction, in certain patients, treating the signs and symptoms of HF may lead to a slower heart rate as the sympathetic surge secondary to breathlessness is mitigated. In contrast, AF may be the inciting cause of HF and thus either slowing the rate or, in certain circumstances, cardioversion, may be the most important goal of therapy. With the exception of patients who are hemodynamically unstable or present with other signs suggesting immediate cardioversion, the approach must be tailored for each patient.

In general, patients with new-onset AHFS secondary to AF should either be cardioverted according to guideline recommendations[45] or rate controlled. If the patient has a history of chronic HF and presents with acute decompensation, the following algorithm may be considered: if the patient is unstable, immediate cardioversion according to guidelines should be considered. If the patient is stable, as a general rule, the use of non-dihydropyridine calcium channel blockers (eg, diltiazem) may be used as per usual management of AF with RVR. In general, β-blockers should not be used.

However, it is the exceptions to these general recommendations that are important. First, is the EF known? Patients with HF and preserved EF may be more dependent on adequate filling or diastole. For these patients, use of either nondihydropyridine calcium channel blockers or short-acting β-blockers (eg, esmolol) is appropriate because there is less concern for any detrimental effects from negative inotropy. If the EF is severely reduced, empirical use of nondihydropyridine calcium channel blockers, which is commonly observed in clinical practice because of their common use in patients with AF and RVR, may have deleterious downstream consequences. Although the rate may be controlled, nondihydropyridine calcium channel blockers such as diltiazem are not short acting, with a half-life of 4 to 6 hours. Thus, the consequences of negative inotropy may be severe. However, these negative downstream effects are often not seen while the patient is in the ED, but remain important considerations. An alternative in this setting, in the absence of concerns for ongoing ischemia, is the use of IV digoxin. Contrary to traditional teaching, the effects of IV digoxin may be seen as early as 30 minutes.[46]

DISPOSITION

Markers of high risk have been well established in HF (**Table 3**). However, the absence of these high-risk features does not equate to a low-risk patient.[47] Who then, is safe to discharge? Given the absence of well-defined prospectively studied guidelines, decisions should be made on an individual basis taking into account not only the patients' clinical status but also their socioeconomic and health literacy, among other considerations. High postdischarge adverse event rates likely now lead to conservative disposition decisions favoring admission. A recent study published from a large administrative database in Canada suggests that patients discharged are at higher risk for postdischarge events than those admitted.[48] Novel approaches to risk stratification are needed and are currently being studied.[47] In the meantime, although not prospectively validated, discharge may be considered for those patients in whom (1) high-risk features are absent during a period of observation, (2) the precipitant for decompensation has been diagnosed and treated, (3) return to baseline compensated state has occurred, (4) a clear and detailed follow-up discharge plan is in place, and (5) physicians' clinical impression is of low risk.

SUMMARY

Post-discharge mortality and morbidity from AHFS are high, affecting nearly half of all discharged patients within 90 days. ED therapy remains largely empiric with minimal evidence to support definitive recommendations to guide therapy. However, lessons learned from recent registries and trials suggests an approach to initial management based on clinical profiles, as defined by high, normal, or low blood pressure. Clinicians are provided with a practical and consensus-driven approach to everyday AHFS management.

REFERENCES

1. Gheorghiade M, Zannad F, Sopko G, et al. Acute heart failure syndromes: current state and framework for future research. Circulation 2005;112(25):3958–68.

2. Lloyd-Jones D, Adams RJ, Brown TM, et al. Heart disease and stroke statistics–2010 update: a report from the American Heart Association. Circulation 2010; 121(7):e46–215.

3. Jencks SF, Williams MV, Coleman EA. Rehospitalizations among patients in the Medicare fee-for-service program. N Engl J Med 2009;360(14):1418–28.

4. Gheorghiade M, Abraham WT, Albert NM, et al. Systolic blood pressure at admission, clinical characteristics, and outcomes in patients hospitalized with acute heart failure. JAMA 2006;296(18):2217–26.

5. Pang PS, Komajda M, Gheorghiade M. The current and future management of acute heart failure syndromes. Eur Heart J 2010;31(7):784–93.

6. Hunt SA, Abraham WT, Chin MH, et al. 2009 Focused update incorporated into the ACC/AHA 2005 guidelines for the diagnosis and management of heart failure in adults: a report of the American College of Cardiology Foundation/American Heart Association Task Force on Practice Guidelines developed in collaboration with the International Society for Heart and Lung Transplantation. J Am Coll Cardiol 2009;53(15):e1–90.

7. Roger VL, Go AS, Lloyd-Jones DM, et al. Heart disease and stroke statistics–2011 update: a report from the American Heart Association. Circulation 2011; 123(4):e18–209.

8. Fonarow GC. The Acute Decompensated Heart Failure National Registry (ADHERE): opportunities to improve care of patients hospitalized with acute decompensated heart failure. Rev Cardiovasc Med 2003;4(Suppl 7):S21–30.

9. Adams KF Jr, Fonarow GC, Emerman CL, et al. Characteristics and outcomes of patients hospitalized for heart failure in the United States: rationale, design, and preliminary observations from the first 100,000 cases in the Acute Decompensated Heart Failure National Registry (ADHERE). Am Heart J 2005;149(2): 209–16.

10. Fonarow GC, Stough WG, Abraham WT, et al. Characteristics, treatments, and outcomes of patients with preserved systolic function hospitalized for heart failure: a report from the OPTIMIZE-HF Registry. J Am Coll Cardiol 2007;50(8):768–77.

11. Fonarow GC, Adams KF Jr, Abraham WT, et al. Risk stratification for in-hospital mortality in acutely decompensated heart failure: classification and regression tree analysis. JAMA 2005;293(5):572–80.

12. Gheorghiade M, Konstam MA, Burnett JC Jr, et al. Short-term clinical effects of tolvaptan, an oral vasopressin antagonist, in patients hospitalized for heart failure: the EVEREST Clinical Status Trials. JAMA 2007;297(12):1332–43.

13. Konstam MA, Gheorghiade M, Burnett JC Jr, et al. Effects of oral tolvaptan in patients hospitalized for worsening heart failure: the EVEREST outcome trial. JAMA 2007;297(12):1319–31.

14. Massie BM, O'Connor CM, Metra M, et al. Rolofylline, an adenosine A1-receptor antagonist, in acute heart failure. N Engl J Med 2010;363(15):1419–28.

15. McMurray JJV, Teerlink JR, Cotter G, et al. Effects of Tezosentan on symptoms and clinical outcomes in patients with acute heart failure: the VERITAS randomized controlled trials. JAMA 2007;298(17):2009–19.

16. Mebazaa A, Nieminen MS, Packer M, et al. Levosimendan vs dobutamine for patients with acute decompensated heart failure: the SURVIVE randomized trial. JAMA 2007;297(17):1883–91.

17. O'Connor CM, Starling RC, Hernandez AF, et al. Effect of nesiritide in patients with acute decompensated heart failure. N Engl J Med 2011;365(1):32–43.

18. Ramirez A, Abelmann WH. Cardiac decompensation. N Engl J Med 1974;290: 499–501.

19. Felker GM, O'Connor CM, Braunwald E, et al. Loop diuretics in acute decompensated heart failure: necessary? Evil? A necessary evil? Circ Heart Fail 2009;2(1):56–62.
20. Gheorghiade M, Pang PS. Acute heart failure syndromes. J Am Coll Cardiol 2009; 53(7):557–73.
21. Pang PS, Cleland JG, Teerlink JR, et al. A proposal to standardize dyspnoea measurement in clinical trials of acute heart failure syndromes: the need for a uniform approach. Eur Heart J 2008;29(6):816–24.
22. Wang CS, FitzGerald JM, Schulzer M, et al. Does this dyspneic patient in the emergency department have congestive heart failure? JAMA 2005;294(15):1944–56.
23. Gheorghiade M, Filippatos G, De Luca L, et al. Congestion in acute heart failure syndromes: an essential target of evaluation and treatment. Am J Med 2006; 119(12 Suppl 1):S3–10.
24. Mahdyoon H, Klein R, Eyler W, et al. Radiographic pulmonary congestion in end-stage congestive heart failure. Am J Cardiol 1989;63(9):625–7.
25. Maisel A, Mueller C, Adams K Jr, et al. State of the art: using natriuretic peptide levels in clinical practice. Eur J Heart Fail 2008;10(9):824–39.
26. Mueller C, Laule-Kilian K, Schindler C, et al. Cost-effectiveness of B-type natriuretic peptide testing in patients with acute dyspnea. Arch Intern Med 2006; 166(10):1081–7.
27. Mueller T, Gegenhuber A, Poelz W, et al. Diagnostic accuracy of B type natriuretic peptide and amino terminal proBNP in the emergency diagnosis of heart failure. Heart 2005;91(5):606–12.
28. Maisel AS, Peacock WF, McMullin N, et al. Timing of immunoreactive B-type natriuretic peptide levels and treatment delay in acute decompensated heart failure: an ADHERE (Acute Decompensated Heart Failure National Registry) analysis. J Am Coll Cardiol 2008;52(7):534–40.
29. Collins S, Storrow AB, Kirk JD, et al. Beyond pulmonary edema: diagnostic, risk stratification, and treatment challenges of acute heart failure management in the emergency department. Ann Emerg Med 2008;51(1):45–57.
30. Dickstein K, Cohen-Solal A, Filippatos G, et al. ESC guidelines for the diagnosis and treatment of acute and chronic heart failure 2008: the Task Force for the Diagnosis and Treatment of Acute and Chronic Heart Failure 2008 of the European Society of Cardiology. Developed in collaboration with the Heart Failure Association of the ESC (HFA) and endorsed by the European Society of Intensive Care Medicine (ESICM). Eur Heart J 2008;29(19):2388–442.
31. Gray A, Goodacre S, Newby DE, et al. Noninvasive ventilation in acute cardiogenic pulmonary edema. N Engl J Med 2008;359(2):142–51.
32. Masip J, Roque M, Sanchez B, et al. Noninvasive ventilation in acute cardiogenic pulmonary edema: systematic review and meta-analysis. JAMA 2005;294(24): 3124–30.
33. ADHERE Scientific Advisory Committee. Acute Decompensated Heart Failure National Registry (ADHERE) core module Q1 2006. Final cumulative national benchmark report. Fremont (CA): Scios Inc; 2006.
34. VMAC Investigators. Intravenous nesiritide vs nitroglycerin for treatment of decompensated congestive heart failure: a randomized controlled trial. JAMA 2002;287(12):1531–40.
35. Peacock WF, Emerman C, Costanzo MR, et al. Early vasoactive drugs improve heart failure outcomes. Congest Heart Fail 2009;15(6):256–64.
36. Cotter G, Metzkor E, Kaluski E, et al. Randomised trial of high-dose isosorbide dinitrate plus low-dose furosemide versus high-dose furosemide plus low-dose isosorbide dinitrate in severe pulmonary oedema. Lancet 1998;351(9100):389–93.

37. Silvers SM, Howell JM, Kosowsky JM, et al. Clinical policy: critical issues in the evaluation and management of adult patients presenting to the emergency department with acute heart failure syndromes. Ann Emerg Med 2007;49(5): 627–69.

38. Swedberg K, Held P, Kjekshus J, et al. Effects of the early administration of enalapril on mortality in patients with acute myocardial infarction. Results of the Cooperative New Scandinavian Enalapril Survival Study II (CONSENSUS II). N Engl J Med 1992;327(10):678–84.

39. Hauptman PJ, Schnitzler MA, Swindle J, et al. Use of nesiritide before and after publications suggesting drug-related risks in patients with acute decompensated heart failure. JAMA 2006;296(15):1877–84.

40. Sackner-Bernstein J, Kowalski M, Fox M, et al. Short-term risk of death after treatment with nesiritide for decompensated heart failure. JAMA 2005;293(15): 1900–5.

41. Sackner-Bernstein JD, Skopicki HA, Aaronson KD. Risk of worsening renal function with nesiritide in patients with acutely decompensated heart failure. Circulation 2005;111(12):1487–91.

42. Peacock WF, Hollander JE, Diercks DB, et al. Morphine for acute decompensated heart failure: valuable adjunct or a historical remnant? Acad Emerg Med 2005; 12(5 Suppl 1):97–8.

43. Peacock WF, Hollander JE, Diercks DB, et al. Morphine and outcomes in acute decompensated heart failure: an ADHERE analysis. Emerg Med J 2008;25(4): 205–9.

44. Peacock WF, Fonarow GC, Ander DS, et al. Society of Chest Pain Centers recommendations for the evaluation and management of the observation stay acute heart failure patient-parts 1-6. Acute Card Care 2009;11(1):3–42.

45. Fuster V, Ryden LE, Cannom DS, et al. ACC/AHA/ESC 2006 guidelines for the management of patients with atrial fibrillation: a report of the American College of Cardiology/American Heart Association Task Force on Practice Guidelines and the European Society of Cardiology Committee for Practice Guidelines (Writing Committee to Revise the 2001 Guidelines for the Management of Patients With Atrial Fibrillation): developed in collaboration with the European Heart Rhythm Association and the Heart Rhythm Society. Circulation 2006;114(7): e257–354.

46. Lanoxin - digoxin injection, solution. PDRNet; 2010. Available at: www.pdr.net. Accessed January 25, 2010.

47. Collins SP, Storrow AB. Acute heart failure risk stratification: can we define low risk? Heart Fail Clin 2009;5(1):75–83, vii.

48. Lee DS, Schull MJ, Alter DA, et al. Early deaths in heart failure patients discharged from the emergency department: a population-based analysis. Circ Heart Fail 2010;3(2):228–35.

Acute Coronary Syndrome Clinical Presentations and Diagnostic Approaches in the Emergency Department

Maame Yaa A.B. Yiadom, MD, MPH

KEYWORDS

- Acute coronary syndrome • Chest pain
- Cardiac biomarkers • Cardiac ischemia

A 47-year-old woman with a history of gastroesophageal reflux disease, hypertension, and hyperlipidemia arrives in the emergency department complaining of shortness of breath for 4 hours. It began abruptly and is accompanied by nausea and vomiting. She has had these symptoms before, but they resolved with Maalox and were never this uncomfortable. Her vital signs are normal, she is given a lidocaine and Maalox suspension and zofran, which alleviates her discomfort. Her electrocardiogram, basic laboratory studies, and troponin sent on arrival are normal. Two hours later she looks and feels well. She is discharged home with a diagnosis of noncardiac chest pain and reflux disease exacerbation. Seven hours later, she returns to the emergency department poorly responsive with an electrocardiogram diagnostic of a ST-elevation myocardial infarction. In the coronary catheterization laboratory she is found to have a fully occlusive lesion in her left anterior descending artery.

Many discussions of cardiac ischemia start with chest pain. It is a chief complaint that captures attention because it is one of the most common emergency department (ED) patient presenting complaints, and is associated with potential life-threatening diagnoses, such as acute coronary syndrome (ACS), pulmonary embolism, and aortic dissection. However, the identification of cardiac ischemia, as is captured within the spectrum of ACS, requires one to cast a broader net. There are now years of research showing that nonclassic ACS symptoms (eg, shortness of breath, fatigue, and nausea)

This author has nothing to disclose.
Department of Emergency Medicine, The Cooper Heart Institute, Robert Wood Johnson Medical School, Cooper University Hospital, 1 Cooper Plaza, Camden, NJ 08103, USA
E-mail address: myiadom@gmail.com

Emerg Med Clin N Am 29 (2011) 689–697
doi:10.1016/j.emc.2011.08.006
0733-8627/11/$ – see front matter © 2011 Elsevier Inc. All rights reserved.

are common and do not reflect less severe disease.[1–4] These are the patients in whom a diagnosis of ACS is likely to be missed,[5] and the biggest medicolegal risk as a specialty.[6,7] There were 124 million United States ED visits in 2010.[8] It is challenging to identify the 16% that will have ACS, particularly when the symptoms are more subtle.[9]

ACS CONTINUUM

ACS is a specific physiology that results in myocardial injury where a thrombus forms on an acutely ruptured acute coronary artery wall to heal the defect. If this clot obstructs the artery's lumen, it can diminish blood flow to tissues beyond the lesion. Diminished flow leads myocardial ischemia, or the process of cells starving for oxygen and other nutrients delivered by the blood.[10] When this process leads to cells starving to death, myocardial infarction occurs and myocardial cell components are released into the blood. The experience of injury from this physiology is represented by three clinical entities: (1) ST-elevation myocardial infarction (STEMI), (2) non-ST elevation myocardial infarction (NSTEMI), and (3) unstable angina (UA). Acute myocardial infarction (AMI) is a subset of ACS that includes both STEMI and NSTEMI.

STEMI is the most urgent and severe condition within ACS. It represents a complete occlusion of a coronary artery leading to full-thickness myocardial infarction, and its diagnosis is based solely on the presence of ST segment elevation on the electrocardiogram (ECG) that meets specific STEMI criteria.[11,12] NSTEMI represents myocardial cell loss and can be identified either by ECG changes or a positive biomarker evaluation, which typically consists of two samples of cardiac enzymes where one is drawn on arrival and the other hours later.[13] The diagnosis of UA is a clinical diagnosis made based on the report of symptom quality and duration. It represents a patient with known coronary disease (CAD) causing a coronary flow limitation who reports a recent history of symptoms that are accelerating or induced with less activity. Also included in this category are patients without a history of angina or CAD who are presenting with a report of symptoms concerning for ischemia without evidence of myocardial cell infarction. These patients are at risk for AMI and can evolve to have a NSTEMI or STEMI. The diagnosis of UA can only be confirmed in the setting of normal or unchanged ECGs, and a negative biomarker evaluation. Until this occurs NSTEMI should be included as the potential diagnosis.[14]

Cardiac biomarkers, typically troponin and creatine kinase-MB (CKMB) levels, serve as tests for myocardial injury. When ACS is suspected, signs of acute myocardial injury are assumed to be from ischemia-caused infarction, or primary (Type I) ACS.[15] However, this is not always a direct relationship. Myocardial injury may be the consequence of another medical condition stressing the heart. This is often referred to as "demand ischemia" (Type II ACS). In addition, other myocardial injury mechanisms, such as direct trauma and surgical manipulation, can elevate serum troponin levels. False elevations can occur because of poor serum troponin clearance, as often seen in end-stage renal disease patients.

Early treatment of ACS is the essential element in reducing morbidity and mortality. Because cardiac biomarker results have become available within the time frame of an ED evaluation, the burden of diagnosis, treatment, and mobilization of definitive therapy is a focus of emergency medical care. One approach to reducing the frequency of missed AMI is to test patients more liberally. However, this poses two problems. First, any test's negative predictive value and positive predictive value are dependent on the prevalence of disease in the test population. If those without concerning symptoms receive the test, its usefulness is reduced.[16] Second, this approach does not take into account the need for appropriate resource use in an era where cost containment is a priority and value-added diagnostics are encouraged and increasingly monitored.

There are robust guidelines providing evidence-based recommendations for the management of patients with ACS and their care. The most widely endorsed are those of the American Heart Association and European Cardiology Associations joint recommendations for STEMI[11] and NSTEM/UA.[13] However, the hardest parts of ACS diagnosis and treatments in the ED are the least informed with clinical evidence. Specifically these challenges are identifying patients whose symptoms may be caused by ACS, and deciding which patients are safe to send home from the ED after what type and extent of testing. The data supporting such decision making are growing, and are discussed in this article.

PATIENT SCREENING FOR POTENTIAL ACS

The ECG is often described as the front-line screening tool for ACS. Altered ion channel function in ischemic tissue can change the electrical conduction pattern, and ECGs can often detect these electrical abnormalities. The ECG is one of the earliest cardiac diagnostic technologies,[17] and this history has made it a hallmark tool in the identification of ACS. However, the criteria for a good screening test or examination is that it has high sensitivity and high specificity,[18] and the ECG has very poor sensitivity, being normal in more than 5% to 10% of all patients eventually diagnosed with AMI, and normal or nondiagnostic (nonspecific ST or T-wave changes) in more than 50% in those with a missed MI.[2]

The Clinical History

The true screening tool is the clinical history. The patient's prior medical history helps gauge their demographic risk. Because CAD is a predisposing condition for ACS, considering a patient's Framingham risk factors (age >55, male gender, diabetic, hypertension, hyperlipidemia, smoker, or family history of an early CAD in a first-degree relative)[19] or TIMI score[20] is helpful in assessing the likelihood that the patient falls into a population of patients with a higher incidence of CAD. However, presenting to an ED with chest pain or other ACS-associated symptoms is more predictive of disease than demographic risk factors.[21] Demographic risk is a reflection of population risk, which is helpful for general risk stratification. It is important to note that in the rare cases of missed ACS these patients are more often non-white, female, or less than 45 years of age. However, it is less important when assessing the incident risk, or whether a particular presentation in a patient is likely to be ACS. A better assessment of risk for ACS is the story behind the patient's arrival in the ED.

The first clinical decision point is whether one believes the complex of symptoms leading up to the clinical encounter could be accounted for by ACS. This is an assessment of the patient's incident risk. Conventional teaching differentiates between classic or typical symptoms (chest pain or crushing pressure, radiating discomfort to the right shoulder and arm [highly specific], the left shoulder and arm, with jaw or neck pain) from atypical symptoms (pricking or stabbing chest pain, shortness of breath, fatigue, dizziness, nausea, upper abdominal pain). Classic symptoms are more specific of ACS, whereas atypical symptoms are less specific given that they have more significant overlap with other diagnoses.[2] However, atypical symptoms are not infrequent or a sign of less severe disease. They account for anywhere between 20% and 30% of all patients with ACS.[2,5] Certain populations, such as women, the elderly, and diabetics, are more likely to present with atypical symptoms and may never have chest pain.[2,20,22] Many patients who end up with coronary revascularization never experienced chest pain.

The ECG

Once the decision is made to evaluate the patient for potential ACS, the ECG is the first, oldest, and fastest test. It is recommended that any patient with symptoms concerning for potential ACS have an ECG performed within 10 minutes to evaluate for potential STEMI, which requires rapid identification and management. The reality of ED patient flow is that patients rarely make it through registration and triage within 10 minutes. Individual EDs need to devise ways to meet this goal in parallel with patient check-in procedures. Methods have included nursing triage protocols identifying patients who should have an early ECGs performed, performing an EKG on arrival for every patient who has a chief complaint involving an organ system from the clavicle to the umbilicus, and direct-to-room triage of all patients for early provider evaluation.

ECGs have limited sensitivity and specificity, so they cannot be used to rule out ACS alone. In addition, they are a single snapshot of a dynamic process.[23] A patient with a normal ECG may evolve into an NSTEMI or STEMI, and some NSTEMIs can become a STEMI with time. Repeating ECG within reasonable intervals to assess for change provides a more longitudinal data. In addition, dynamic ST segment and T-wave changes should increase one's concern for AMI.[24]

The Physical Examination

Signs of heart failure can be a consequence of ischemia. However, the physical examination adds little to the identification of ACS directly. It is helpful in exploring the likelihood of conditions within the differential diagnosis for ACS symptoms. These include pneumonia, aortic dissection, pulmonary embolism, pneumothorax, musculoskeletal pain, pericardial effusion, and reflux disease.

Cardiac Biomarkers

In light of the limited diagnostic capabilities of the ECG, biomarker testing is an essential part of making the diagnosis. There are many biomarkers available with which to detect ischemia. These include myoglobin, CKMB, and cardiac troponins T or I.[14] In the 1990s, CKMB and the associated CKMB/total CK ratio were the gold standard for AMI diagnosis. They are still widely used, but have been replaced by cardiac-specific troponin T and I as the gold standard. Troponins are more sensitive tests for myocardial ischemia, but early generation troponins were found to have levels detectable in serum 4 to 12 hours after symptom onset (**Fig. 1**).

As a result CKMB, which is present in serum and reaches peak levels earlier than troponin, is still used in many facilities as an early warning test.[25] However, it is not recommended for making a final diagnosis of AMI if troponin testing is available.[12] Data from two recent studies indicate that this early warning value for CKMB testing may not be needed with new third- and fourth-generation troponin assays: ultrasensitive troponin I and troponin T. Troponins were elevated much earlier using these highly sensitive assays, obviating any need for CK measurements.[26,27]

Cardiac biomarkers are a direct test for myocardial injury, and ACS is one of many processes that lead to myocardial injury; thus, elevated troponin level does not always indicate AMI. In the absence of an alternative diagnosis a positive troponin should be assumed to be evidence of myocardial infarction until proved otherwise. A recent study noted that most troponin elevations in ED patients are from noncardiac causes and that a hospital discharge diagnosis of primary AMI was assigned to only 11% of patients admitted with positive troponin values.[28] If an alternative diagnosis exists, the

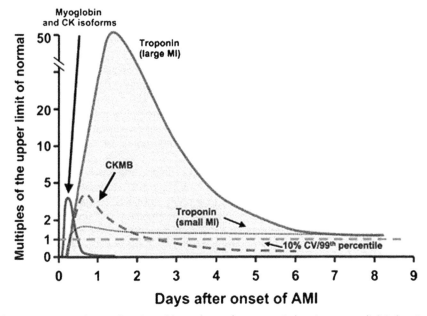

Fig. 1. Time to release of various biomarkers after acute ischemic myocardial infarction. (*From* Anderson JL, Adams CD, Antman EM, et al. ACC/AHA 2007 guidelines for the management of patients with unstable angina/non–ST-Elevation myocardial infarction. J Am Coll Cardiol 2007;50(7):e26; with permission.)

possibility of AMI as a cause or consequence of that condition should be considered against a troponin elevation from an alternative mechanism of myocardial injury. If it is unclear, AMI should be treated and the course re-evaluated with time, repeat biomarkers, and consideration of a cardiology consultation. Examples of the latter case include atrial fibrillation with a rapid ventricular response that could be a consequence of primary ischemia or the cause of secondary ischemia because of the excessive cardiac demand of the tachycardia. Also, patients with an abnormal troponin level caused by a non-AMI source often have a worse prognosis than if they had had an AMI, and therefore should be admitted.

EXTENT OF TESTING

No test or work-up is perfect. This makes missed cases an expectation. However, there is no acceptable miss rate for ACS. Recent studies have demonstrated rates of 2% to 3%. But most were done before the era of ultrasensitive troponins. It is expected that the more sensitive assays have improved case capture, but the miss rate with current practice is still unclear. Similarly, it is not known what degree of investment and additional testing will reduce this number. The impact of observation medicine and emergent stress testing on miss rates is not directly known. Despite this data void, figuring out how much testing to do for which patients is an active clinical question faced multiple times a day by emergency and family medicine physicians, internists, and cardiologists.

It is encouraged to use the clinical history (demographic risk and incident risk) and ECG to risk stratify patients for the likelihood of ACS. One should use caution when using these three items to rule out cardiac chest pain in moderate- and high-risk patients. When the history and ECG alone are used to formulate a diagnostic impression of noncardiac chest pain, 2% to 5% of ACS cases are missed.[29,30] Having a higher demographic risk profile (CAD, prior myocardial infarction, multiple CAD risk factors, and so forth) was correlated with missed events (**Table 1**).[31]

For patients with lower-risk profiles, most specifically those who have had a limited lifetime to acquire CAD, ACS is less prevalent. Mason and colleagues[32] found that missed ACS rates were less than 0.14% among non–cocaine using patients with symptoms concerning for ACS who have no CAD history, are less than 40 years of age, without CAD risk factors or a normal ECG, and a negative initial set of biomarkers. This work-up can be considered in these lower demographic risk patients when their incident risk is believe to be low.

In cases of missed AMI, the usefulness of ECG in diagnosing AMI is limited by physician ECG interpretation. Key pitfalls include interpreting ST depressions as a strain rather than evidence of NSTEMI, failure to identify subtle ST segment elevations, not recognizing nonspecific ST and T-wave abnormalities as signs of potential ischemia, and not pursuing ischemia as a cause of new bundle branch blocks.[1,6,7]

If the decision is made to further pursue potential ACS, there are several tools available. First is to extend the evaluation for AMI by repeating the cardiac biomarkers after a time interval. When to repeat the biomarkers is highly dependent on the onset of symptoms, the biomarkers positive and negative predictive value, the kinetics of release, and clearance in the serum. The sensitivity, positive productive values of troponin, is greater than CKMB, and CKMB's performance in these areas is greater than myoglobin. It is generally accepted to repeat an older-generation troponin within 8 to 12 hours and a newer-generation troponin within 6 to 9 hours.[33,34] Current international guidelines recommend testing at presentation and at 6 hours. However, new data suggest that newer troponin assays may be reliable at as few as 3 hours, although there is no study that supports making disposition decisions using these new assays at any interval.[26,27]

Table 1
Screening and early diagnostic tools for acute coronary syndrome

Tools	Pretest Probability		ACS Early Diagnostic Tools	
	Demographic Risk	Incident Risk	ECG	Cardiac Enzyme
	CAD risk factors	Typical Symptoms	ST segment elevations that meet STEMI criteria or a new LBBB	Elevated troponin
	Diabetes	Chest pain, pressure or discomfort		Normal troponin but an elevated CKMB ratio
	Hypertension	Arm pain		
	Hyperlipidemia	Neck/jaw pain		
	Smoking	Atypical symptoms	ST elevations that do not meet STEMI criteria	Normal troponin and normal CKMB ratio
	Family history of early CAD in a first-degree relative	Shortness of breath	New ST depressions	Elevated CKMB with a Normal CKMB ratio only
		Fatigue	New T-wave inversion in a coronary distribution	
	Age >45 for men or >55 for women	Nausea		
		Vomiting		
		Dizziness		
	Male gender	Upper abdominal pain	ST and T-wave abnormalities in a nonspecific (noncoronary) distribution	
			Normal ECG	

If this testing is negative, the next step is to consider potential UA, by testing for reproducible ischemia with exercise testing or nuclear stress testing. The most common modalities are exercise treadmill testing, sestamibi scanning, and stress echocardiography. These tests were not initially developed for UA evaluations in patients without a history of prior CAD or myocardial infarction, but their use is becoming common in hospitals, chest pain units, and directly from many EDs. Their positive predictive value, as with most tests, is dependent on the prevalence of disease in the risk population, so when a test is positive in a low-risk patient it is more likely to be a false-positive. However, their negative predictive value for 30-day adverse events approaches 100% when a structured interpretation (eg, the Duke score) is used. The reverse is true in high-risk patients.[35] For the low-risk ED patient, the clinical yield of these provocative tests on reducing missed ACS has not yet been demonstrated. Evolving literature in this area is sure to comment in coming years.

Another method of extending the ACS evaluation is to look for the presence or absence of a flow-limiting lesion or CAD. This is a well-established approach used in higher-risk patients when they can be admitted for coronary catheterization. In very-low-risk patients coronary CT angiography is emerging as a noninvasive means of ruling out ACS by demonstrating the lack of a flow-limiting lesion or CAD. Whether the goal of an ED visit should be to evaluate for CAD in this population is up for debate. However, in patients with a low likelihood for coronary disease, ruling out CAD can help clinicians to pursue other etiologies of pain, if the presenting story is concerning and the ECGs and biomarker testing are negative. The radiation involved is approximately 50% to 75% less than an abdominal CT scan.

All patients evaluated for CAD with negative testing should be given very clear discharge instructions with details on when to return for re-evaluation. Setting up a very specific primary care or cardiology follow-up plan creates a safety net for potentially missed disease.

REFERENCES

1. Pope JH, Aufderheide TP, Ruthazer R, et al. Missed diagnosis of acute cardiac ischemia in the emergency department. N Engl J Med 2000;342: 1163–70.
2. Mehta RH, Eagle KA. Missed diagnosis of acute coronary syndrome in the emergency room: continuing challenges. N Engl J Med 2000;342(16): 1207–9.
3. Zucker DR, Griffith JL, Beshansky JR, et al. Presentations of acute myocardial infarction in men and women. J Gen Intern Med 1997;12:79–87.
4. Lusiani L, Perrone A, Pesavento R, et al. Prevalence, clinical features and acute course of atypical myocardial infarction. Angiology 1994;45(1):49–55.
5. Pope JH, Selker HP. Diagnosis of acute cardiac ischemia. Emerg Med Clin North Am 2003;21(1):27–59.
6. Karcz A, Korn R, Burke MC, et al. Malpractice claims against emergency physicians in Massachusetts: 1975–1993. Am J Emerg Med 1996;14:341–5.
7. Rusnak RA, Stair TO, Hansen K, et al. Litigation against the emergency physician: common features in cases of missed myocardial infarction. Ann Emerg Med 1989; 18:1029–34.
8. Garcia TC, Bernstein AB, Bush MA. Emergency department visitors and visits: who used the emergency room in 2007. NCHS Data Brief 2010;38:1–8.
9. Pitts SR, Niska RW, Xu J. National Hospital Ambulatory Medical Care Summary: 2006. Natl Health Stat Report 2008;(7):1–38.

10. Brady WJ, Harrigan RA, Chan T. Acute coronary syndrome. In: Rosen's emergency medicine: concepts and clinical practice. 6th edition. St Louis: Mosby; 2006. p. 1155–7.
11. Kosowsky JM, Yiadom MY. The diagnosis and treatment of STEMI in the emergency department. Emerg Med Pract 2009;11(6):2.
12. Kushner FG, Hand M, Smith SC Jr, et al. 2009 focused update: ACC/AHA guidelines for the management of patients with ST-elevation myocardial infarction. J Am Coll Cardiol 2009;54:2205–41.
13. Doshi AA, Iskyan K, Oneil JM, et al. Evaluation and management of non–ST–segment elevation acute coronary syndromes in the emergency department. Emerg Med Pract 2010;12(1):1–25.
14. Anderson JL, Adams CD, Fletcher RW, et al. ACC/AHA 2007 guidelines for the management of patients with unstable angina/non–ST-elevation myocardial infarction. J Am Coll Cardiol 2007;50:e1–157.
15. Thygesen K, Alpert JS, White HD, et al. Universal definition of myocardial infarction. Eur Heart J 2007;28:2527–38.
16. Altman DG. Statistics note: diagnostic tests 2: predictive values. BMJ 1994; 309(102):1.
17. Waller AD. A demonstration on man of electromotive changes accompanying the heart's beat. J Physiol (Lond) 1887;8:229–34.
18. Fletcher RW, Fletcher SW. Clinical epidemiology: the essentials. Philadelphia: Lippincott; 2005.
19. Gordon T, Sorlie P, Kannel W. Atherothrombotic brain infarction, intermittent claudication. A multivariate coronary head disease analysis of some factors related to their incidence: Framingham Study, 16 years follow up. Washington, DC: US Government Printing Office; 1971.
20. Hess EP, Agarwal D, Chandra S, et al. Diagnostic accuracy of the TIMI risk score in patients with chest pain in the emergency department: a meta-analysis. CMAJ 2010;182(10):1039–44.
21. Jayes RL, Beshansky JR, D'Agostino RB, et al. Do patients' coronary risk factor reports predict acute cardiac ischemia in the emergency department? J Clin Epidemiol 1992;45(6):621–6.
22. Canto JG, Goldbert RJ, Hand MM. Symptom presentations of women with acute coronary syndrome. The Female Patient: Women's Heart Health. Vol 25, March 2009. Available at: http://www.femalepatient.com/PDF/034030026.pdf. Accessed August 2, 2011.
23. Herring N, Paterson DJ. ECG diagnosis of acute ischaemia and infarction past, present and future. QJM 2006;99:219–30.
24. Rautaharjo PM, Surawicz B, Gettes LS. AHA/ACCF/HRS recommendations for the standardization and interpretation of electrocardiogram: part IV: the ST segment, T and U waves, and QT interval. Circulation 2009;119:e241–50.
25. Morrow DA, Cannon CP, Jesse RL. National academy of clinical biochemistry laboratory medicine practice guidelines: clinical characteristics and utilization of biochemical markers in acute coronary syndromes. Circulation 2007;115:e356–75.
26. Selker T, Zeller T, Peetz D, et al. Sensitive troponin I assay in early diagnosis of acute myocardial infarction. N Engl J Med 2009;361:868–77.
27. Reichlin T, Hochholzer W, Bassetti S, et al. Early diagnosis of myocardial infarction with sensitive cardiac troponin assays. N Engl J Med 2009;361:858.
28. Yiadom MY, Kosowsky JM, Melanson SL, et al. Diagnostic performance of a highly sensitive cardiac troponin I assay in an emergency department setting. Clinical Chemistry 2010;56(Suppl 6):A131.

29. Miller CD, Lindsell CJ, Kandelwal S, et al. Is the initial diagnostic impression of "non cardiac chest pain" adequate to exclude cardiac disease. Ann Emerg Med 2004;3:565–74.
30. Amsterdam EA, Kirk JD, Bluemke AD, et al. Testing of low-risk patients presenting to the emergency department with chest pain. Circulation 2010;122:1756–76.
31. Farkouh ME, Aneja A, Reeder GS, et al. Clinical risk stratification in the emergency department predicts long-term cardiovascular outcomes in a population-based cohort presenting with acute chest pain: primary results of the Olmstead County chest pain study. Medicine 2009;88:307–13.
32. Mason RJ, Shaver KJ, Sease KL, et al. Evaluation for a clinical decision rule for young adult patients with chest pain. Acad Emerg Med 2004;8(42):26–31.
33. O'Connor RE, Brady W, Brooks SC, et al. Part 10: acute coronary syndrome. 2010 AHA guidelines for cardiopulmonary resuscitation and emergency cardiovascular care. Circulation 2010;122:S791.
34. Fesmire FM, Percy RF, Bardoner JB, et al. Serial CKMB testing during emergency department evaluation of chest pain: the utility of a 2 hr change in CKMB of +1.6ng/ml. Am Heart J 1998;136:237–94.
35. Lindsay J Jr, Bunnet YD, Pines EE. Routine stress testing for the triage of patients with chest pain: Is it worth the candle. Ann Emerg Med 1998;32:600–3.

Emergency Department Treatment of Acute Coronary Syndromes

Maame Yaa A.B. Yiadom, MD, MPH

KEYWORDS

- Acute coronary syndrome
- Non-ST-segment elevation myocardial infarction
- ST-segment elevation myocardial infarction
- Non-ST-segment elevation acute coronary syndrome
- Unstable angina • Chest pain • Cardiac ischemia

Acute coronary syndrome (ACS) is a broad term encompassing a spectrum of acute myocardial ischemia and injury ranging from unstable angina (UA) and non–ST-segment elevation myocardial infarction (NSTEMI) to ST-segment elevation myocardial infarction (STEMI). ACS accounts for approximately 1.2 million hospital admissions in the United States annually.[1] The aging of the United States population, along with the national obesity epidemic and the associated increase in metabolic syndrome, means that the number of individuals at risk for ACS will continue to increase for the foreseeable future.[2] This article reviews the current evidence and guidelines for the treatment of patients along the continuum of ACS.

DEFINITIONS

ACS is a syndrome defined by the presence of symptoms, electrocardiographic (ECG) changes, and/or biochemical markers consistent with myocardial ischemia or injury. Typical symptoms include chest pain or pressure, but ACS can also manifest with symptoms such as shortness of breath, nausea, or malaise. ECG changes run the gamut from ST-segment elevations to subtle ST-segment depressions or T-wave inversions. Dynamic ECG changes—those that change or evolve over time—raise particular concern for ACS.[3] In the context of ischemic symptoms, biochemical evidence of myocardial necrosis defines acute myocardial infarction (MI), and the greater the elevation in cardiac biomarkers, the higher the risk of serious morbidity and mortality.

Primary ACS refers to a syndrome of acute myocardial ischemia initiated at the level of the coronary artery itself. The most common form of primary ACS is triggered by

The author has nothing to disclose.
Department of Emergency Medicine, The Cooper Heart Institute, Robert Wood Johnson Medical School, Cooper University Hospital, 1 Cooper Plaza, Camden, NJ 08103, USA
E-mail address: myiadom@gmail.com

Emerg Med Clin N Am 29 (2011) 699–710
doi:10.1016/j.emc.2011.09.016
0733-8627/11/$ – see front matter © 2011 Elsevier Inc. All rights reserved.

emed.theclinics.com

rupture of an atherosclerotic plaque, leading to intraluminal thrombus formation, and either complete or partial occlusion of a coronary artery. The process of coronary thrombus formation is complex. Activation of the coagulation cascade culminates in the production of fibrin, which catalyzes the polymerization of fibrinogen into a fibrin mesh. Platelets adhere and become activated via several receptor-mediated pathways (including the thrombin receptor). Activated platelets express fibrinogen receptors, allowing the aggregation of platelets into the thrombus via fibrin cross-links. Downstream myocardial ischemia and/or injury results directly from the thrombus occluding the coronary blood flow and/or from distal embolization of microthrombi. Less common forms of primary ACS include coronary artery spasm, coronary artery dissection, and coronary artery thromboembolism.

Secondary ACS refers to pathophysiology external to the coronary arteries that precipitates signs and symptoms of coronary ischemia or injury. Any condition that limits myocardial oxygen delivery—profound anemia, hypotension, or hypoxemia, for example—can produce a clinical picture indistinguishable from primary ACS, even in patients with normal coronary anatomy. Just as "supply-side" conditions can precipitate ACS, "demand-side" conditions such as uncontrolled hypertension or tachycardia can create myocardial energy imbalance and lead to ischemia or injury. It may actually be the case that secondary ACS is actually more common than primary ACS, particularly in patients who have underlying coronary artery disease. However, unlike primary ACS, for which management is focused on the coronary thrombus, the approach to secondary ACS is on balancing the supply-demand mismatch by treating the inciting condition, whether it be sepsis, hypovolemia, hypertensive crisis, or tachyarrhythmia.

ST-segment elevation MI (STEMI) is a diagnosis made solely via ECG (**Box 1**). Based on 2007 estimates, STEMI accounts for approximately one-third of all acute MIs.[4] STEMI criteria identifies a subset of ACS patients that benefit from rapid coronary reperfusion therapy.[5] As such, any patient presenting to the emergency department (ED) with symptoms concerning for STEMI should have an ECG done within 10 minutes of arrival.[6]

However, in considering the diagnosis of STEMI, it is also important to note that there are other conditions that may cause ST elevations on an ECG (**Table 1**).

It has been well established that early reperfusion of the infarct-related artery is associated with improved outcome in STEMI.[8] Delay to reperfusion is associated with

---

Box 1
STEMI criteria

American College of Cardiology/American Heart Association ST-Segment Elevation Myocardial Infarction (STEMI) Diagnosis Guidelines[7]
In a patient presenting with active chest pain, a 12-lead electrocardiogram showing:

1. ST-segment elevation $\geq$1 mm (0.1 mV) in 2 or more adjacent limb leads (from aVL to III, including aVR)

2. ST-segment elevation $\geq$1 mm (0.1 mV) in precordial leads V4 through V6

3. ST-segment elevation $\geq$2 mm (0.2 mV) in precordial leads V1 through V3

4. New left bundle-branch block

Therapy should not be delayed while awaiting results or cardiac biomarkers. Reciprocal depressions (ST depressions in the leads corresponding to the opposite side of the heart) make the diagnosis of STEMI more specific.

Table 1
Non-ACS causes of ST-segment elevation

Alternative Diagnosis	Associated History
Benign early repolarization	Young, male, often African American
Coronary vasospasm	Cocaine use, stimulant use, some chemotherapy agents
Left ventricular hypertrophy	Hypertension
Paced rhythm	Implanted pacemaker
Pericarditis/myocarditis	Fevers, recent radiation therapy
Significant hyperkalemia	Renal failure, potassium supplements, digoxin use
Takotsubo cardiomyopathy	Acute, severe emotional stressor
Ventricular aneurysm	Prior MI, active ischemia and NSAID use, recent cardiac surgery

Abbreviations: MI, myocardial infarction; NSAID, nonsteroidal anti-inflammatory drugs.
Data from Slater DK, Hlatky MA, Mark DB, et al. Outcomes in suspected acute myocardial infarction with normal or minimally abnormal admission electrocardiographic findings. Am J Cardiol 1987;60(10):766–70; and Brady WJ, Homer A. Clinical decision-making in adult chest pain patients with electrocardiographic ST-segment elevation: STEMI versus Non-AMI causes of ST-segment abnormality. Emerg Med Prac 2006;8(1):4.

a corresponding increase in STEMI-related mortality. The American Heart Association/American College of Cardiology (AHA/ACC) recommendations establish the standard of care in this regard: ED arrival to fibrinolysis ("door-to-needle" time) within 30 minutes; and an ED arrival to percutaneous coronary intervention (PCI) ("door-to-balloon" time) within 90 minutes.[1]

Non–ST-segment elevation acute coronary syndrome (NSTE-ACS) is a term used to denote ACS not meeting ECG criteria for STEMI. It includes non–ST elevation MI (NSTEMI) and UA. If biomarkers for myonecrosis are positive, the diagnosis of NSTEMI can be made. If not, the clinical syndrome is termed UA. From a clinical standpoint, without a series of cardiac biomarkers for myocardial necrosis (which can take several hours before becoming positive), a distinction between UA and NSTEMI cannot be made (**Fig. 1**).

Other Causes of Myocardial Necrosis

ACS is one of many mechanisms for myocardial cell injury and necrosis, and not all biomarker elevations represent cardiac ischemia. Myocardial cell death can be seen in a wide range of conditions, including acute myocarditis, blunt trauma, chronic cardiomyopathies, drug toxicity, and sepsis.

INITIAL TREATMENT

In some ways, the principles of therapy for all ACSs are fundamentally similar. The common treatment objectives are to:

1. Balance myocardial supply and demand
2. Limit thrombus formation: antiplatelet and anticoagulant therapies
3. Restore lumen patency: angioplasty, stent placement, and coronary artery bypass grafting (CABG).

What distinguishes STEMI from most NSTE-ACS is the urgency and speed with which myocardial blood flow must be restored to prevent irreversible transmural damage, hence the emphasis on rapid reperfusion therapy.

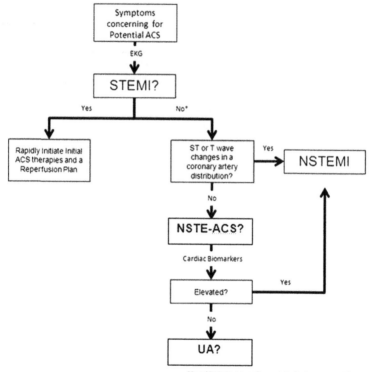

Fig. 1. Making the diagnosis. ACS, acute coronary syndrome; EKG, electrocardiography; NSTE, non–ST-segment elevation; NSTEMI, non–ST-segment elevation myocardial infarction; STEMI, ST-segment elevation myocardial infarction; UA, unstable angina.

Antiplatelet Therapy

All patients with suspected ACS should receive 162 to 325 mg of aspirin as close to the onset of symptoms as possible. Aspirin blocks platelet activation by limiting thromboxane production via the cyclooxygenase pathway. In the absence of reperfusion therapy, aspirin alone provides a near 25% reduction in mortality.[9] Ideally aspirin should be chewed for rapid absorption and effect. If a patient is unable to take medications orally, aspirin can be administered via rectal suppository with an adjusted dose range of 300 to 600 mg. Peak serum levels are reached within 30 minutes with oral dosing and 90 minutes with rectal dosing.[10] For patients with an aspirin allergy, a loading dose of clopidogrel should be given as an alternative. The recommended dose is 300 to 600 mg.[11]

Oxygen

Providing supplemental oxygen is routine practice. However, in patients with normal oxygen saturations, the carrying capacity of their blood hemoglobin and soluble serum oxygen concentration is only minimally affected by increased concentrations of inhaled oxygen. Administering supplemental oxygen is the standard of care for any patient with demonstrated hypoxia, but is considered reasonable in any patient with ACS within in the first 6 hours of presentation.[1,12]

Nitroglycerin

Nitroglycerin (NTG) is considered a reasonable initial therapy for chest pain due to ACS. However, administration of nitrates confers no demonstrated survival benefit with NSTE-ACS,[13] or with STEMI in the context of current reperfusion intervention.[14] Patients can be given 0.4 mg sublingual NTG every 5 minutes, or a continuous intravenous infusion of NTG at a dose of 10 to 50 μg/min. Because of its preload reducing effects, NTG is contraindicated in patients with critical aortic stenosis, and should be used with caution in patients suspected of having right ventricular acute MI. Nitrates are also contraindicated in patients who have used sildenafil within 24 hours (or up to 72 hours with longer-acting phosphodiesterase type 5 inhibitors).

Morphine

Morphine is a reasonable second-line agent for relieving chest pain in patients with ACS in whom nitrates are either contraindicated or fail to eliminate pain.[1] Retrospective data suggest higher morbidity among NSTE-ACS patients receiving morphine,[15] but a causal link is far from established.

β-Blockers

The administration of β-blockers to STEMI patients has been shown to reduce rates of recurrent ischemia and reinfarction following reperfusion therapy.[16] However, routine up-front administration of β-blockers to patients may lead to increased incidence of cardiogenic shock and may outweigh the benefits.[17] Current guidelines recommend against routine intravenous administration of β-blocker for acute STEMI.[18] For NSTE-ACS patients an oral β-blocker should be started within 24 hours of presentation. In all cases, β-blockers should be avoided when there are signs of congestive heart failure, evidence of a low cardiac output state, or other relative contraindications to β-blockade (PR interval >0.24 seconds, second- or third-degree heart block, active asthma, or reactive airway disease).

ST-ELEVATION MYOCARDIAL INFARCTION

The imperative to provide reperfusion therapy as early as possible cannot be overstated. It is generally accepted that all else being equal, primary PCI is preferable to fibrinolytic therapy, in terms of both success in establishing reperfusion and minimizing the risk of hemorrhagic complications. In practice, the choice between fibrinolytic therapy and PCI depends largely on the availability of PCI, such that if primary PCI is not available within 90 minutes of patient arrival, fibrinolytic therapy should be considered.[19] The decision to proceed with fibrinolytic therapy should only occur after consideration of any contraindications (**Table 2**), and should also take into account the duration of symptoms. Fibrinolysis has been shown to have limited success when initiated beyond 3 hours from symptom onset.[20,21] If a patient is not at a PCI-capable facility, transfer should be coordinated ideally within the 90 minute door-to-needle time frame (**Fig 2**).

Once the decision is made to perform PCI, the selection and timing of anticoagulation and antiplatelet adjuncts should be discussed with the receiving interventional cardiologist. For patients receiving fibrinolysis the choices for adjunctive therapy are outlined below.

Facilitated PCI

It has been hypothesized that the early administration of fibrinolytics will "facilitate" the success of eventual PCI. Studies examining the use of full-dose fibrinolytics have

Table 2
Efficacy and risk of common fibrinolytic agents

	Alteplase (tPA or Activase)	Tenecteplase (TNKase)	Reteplase (Retavase)
Reperfusion rate by 90 minutes	79	80	80
Lives saved per 100 persons treated	3.5	3.5	3.0
Risk of intracranial hemorrhage	0.6%	0.5–0.7%	0.8%

Data from Refs.[27–30]

shown greater complications and morbidity.[22] Partial-dose fibrinolytics with a variety of combinations with high-dose heparin and glycoprotein IIb/IIIa (GPIIb/IIIa) inhibitors have shown no improvement in outcomes and in some cases have increased bleeding risk.[19,23] Current guidelines do not support using full-dose fibrinolytics in STEMI patients. However, in moderate-risk and high-risk patients for whom PCI is the ideal strategy, and transport times are prolonged but PCI can be achieved within 2 hours, using partial-dose fibrinolytics may be considered in discussion with the receiving interventional cardiologist (see **Fig. 2**).[19]

If fibrinolysis is planned as primary therapy, the patient must first be screened for risk of the life-threatening hemorrhage (**Box 2**). The most feared complication of fibrinolytic therapy is intracranial hemorrhage (ICH), which occurs with an incidence of 0.6% to 1%,[24] and a mortality rate of about 50%.[25] Risk factors for fibrinolytic-associated ICH include advanced age and uncontrolled hypertension.

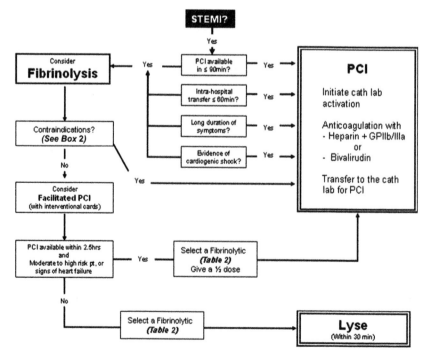

Fig. 2. Choosing between fibrinolytic therapy and percutaneous coronary intervention (PCI) for STEMI patients.

Box 2
Contraindications to fibrinolytic therapy

A. Absolute Contraindications

Known structural central nervous system lesion (eg, arteriovenous malformation, primary or metastatic tumor)

Any prior intracerebral hemorrhage

Ischemic stroke within the last 3 months (excluding acute ischemic stroke within the last 3 hours)

Significant closed head or facial injury within the last 3 months

Suspicion of aortic dissection

Active bleeding (excluding menses) or bleeding disorders

B. Relative Contraindications

History of chronic, severe, and poorly controlled hypertension or severe hypertension (systolic blood pressure >180 mm

Hg or diastolic blood pressure >100 mm Hg on admission

History of ischemic stroke within the prior 3 months

Dementia or other known intracranial pathology not noted above

Traumatic or prolonged (>10 minutes) cardiopulmonary resuscitation or noncompressible vascular punctures within the last 3 weeks

Major surgery within the last 3 weeks

Internal bleeding within the last 3–4 weeks

Pregnancy

Active peptic ulcer disease

Current use of anticoagulants (the higher the international normalized ratio, the greater the risk of bleeding)

Prior exposure (>5 days) or prior allergic reaction to streptokinase or antistreplase (if taking these agents)

Data from Rogers VL, Go AS, Lloyd-Jones DM, et al. Heart disease and stroke statistics—2011 update: a report from the American Heart Association. Circulation 2011;123:e18–209; and Antman EM, Anbe DT, Armstrong PW, et al. ACC/AHA Guidelines for the management of patients with ST-elevation myocardial infarction: executive summary: a report of the American College of Cardiology/American Heart Association Task Force on Practice Guidelines. Circulation 2004;110(5):588–636.

Four fibrinolytic agents have been approved by the Food and Drug Administration for the treatment of STEMI. Selection of one agent over another generally occurs at an institutional level. Streptokinase, the first fibrinolytic, is no longer available in many institutions because of the risk of antibody formation and an immune reaction with exposure or reexposure to the drug. A comparison of the characteristics of various agents is shown in **Table 2**.

Follow-Up PCI

Routine PCI immediately following fibrinolytic administration has not been shown to improve outcomes.[26] However, coronary perfusion following fibrinolytic therapy may be inadequate in up to one-third of cases, as evidenced by persistent ischemic symptoms, failure to see ST-segment resolution, hemodynamic instability, or refractory electrical arrhythmias, and there is proven benefit to intervention with PCI in such cases. Current guidelines recommend an observation period of about 90 minutes, at which point rescue PCI should be considered. Emerging data suggest that routine transfer to a PCI center following fibrinolytic therapy may make sense, so as to facilitate rescue PCI if and when required.

Thienopyridines

This class of antiplatelet agents includes clopidogrel and prasugrel, along with the newly approved ticagrelor. These medications inhibit platelet activation by blocking the adenosine diphosphate receptor. Only ticagrelor binds reversibly, but experience with this drug in the ED is limited. Clopidogrel is the best studied drug in this class and the only one currently approved for administration with fibrinolytic, but it requires the longest time to reach maximal effect. To offset this, loading doses exceeding the usual 300 mg may be given, but caution should be exercised in elderly patients receiving fibrinolytic therapy. Alternatively, for patients undergoing PCI prasugrel may be administered with a loading dose of 60 mg, but patients with a prior history of cerebrovascular disease should not receive prasugrel because of a higher incidence of stroke.

GPIIb/IIIa Inhibitors

This class of intravenous antiplatelet agents, which includes abciximab, eptifibatide, and tirofiban, binds to the fibrinogen receptor to block platelet aggregation. Administration of a GPIIb/IIIa inhibitor at or around the time of primary PCI is standard practice; however, up-front use of GPIIB/IIIa inhibitors before transfer to the catheterization laboratory has not been shown to improve outcomes. For patients in whom a fibrinolytic strategy is selected, there is no demonstrated role for GPIIb/IIIa inhibitors in the ED.

Anticoagulants

For patients in whom a primary PCI strategy is chosen, reasonable choices for adjuvant anticoagulation therapy include unfractionated heparin (UFH), enoxaparin, or bivalirudin. Unfractionated heparin is still the most widely used, and dosing should be weight based. Bivalirudin is an attractive option for PCI because as a more powerful anticoagulant it can obviate the need for GPIIb/IIIa inhibitors and thereby minimize the risk of bleeding. For patients receiving fibrinolytic therapy, UFH and enoxaparin are both reasonable choices. If enoxaparin is chosen, an intravenous loading dose of 60 mg should be administered along with the first subcutaneous dose to patients younger than 75 years. Fondaparinux is an attractive option for patients receiving fibrinolytic therapy who are at high risk of bleeding. Bivalirudin has not been studied as an adjunct to fibrinolytic therapy. For a summary of some of the advantages and disadvantages of various anticoagulants, see **Table 3**.

NON–ST-SEGMENT ELEVATION ACS

For all NSTE-ACS patients, treatment focuses on the stabilization of a partially occlusive thrombus to minimize downstream ischemia and injury, as well as reduce the risk of progression to STEMI. Fibrinolytic therapy has no role, but PCI is increasingly used to prevent recurrent ischemia. In moderate-risk to high-risk cases, early PCI (ie, within 24–72 hours) is associated with improved 30-day outcomes. The precise timing of PCI in NSTE-ACS is dependent, among other things, on the presence of ongoing ischemia and the risk for recurrent ischemia or other cardiovascular morbidity. Risk scores such

Table 3
Anticoagulant therapy options for acute coronary syndrome

Anticoagulant	Pros	Cons	Comparative Bleeding Risk	Expense
Heparin (UFH)	Immediate anticoagulation Easy to monitor Long clinical use history Easy to stop by discontinuing the infusion	Does not inhibit bound thrombin (only free thrombin) Variable anticoagulation effects requiring monitoring	PTT dependent	$
Enoxaparin (LMWH)	More effective thrombin inhibition than UFH Monitoring is not necessary Lower risk of HIT than UFH Long history of clinical use Does not cross the placenta	Does not inhibit bound thrombin (only free thrombin) Less reversible than UFH and bivalirudin Difficult to monitor Renally cleared Long half-life Risk of HIT	Highest	$$
Fondaparinux	Subcutaneous delivery Once-daily dosing Monitoring is not necessary No risk of HIT Does not cross the placenta	Most difficult to monitor Long half-life	Lower	$$$
Bivalirudin	Reduced risk of bleeding No risk of HIT Immediate anticoagulation Easy to stop by discontinuing the infusion	Limited clinical use history Not widely available	Lowest	$$$$

Abbreviations: HIT, heparin-induced thrombocytopenia; LMWH, low molecular weight heparin; PTT, partial thromboplastin time; UFH, unfractionated heparin.
Data from Refs.[31–33]

as TIMI (Thrombolysis in Myocardial Infarction) and GRACE (Global Registry of Acute Coronary Events) have been developed to predict short-term outcomes and define the population of patients most likely to benefit for earlier and more aggressive therapy. Correspondingly, the choice and timing of adjunctive antiplatelet and anticoagulant medications has a lot to do with whether and when PCI is being contemplated.

Patients at highest risk include those with refractory anginal pain, evolving ECG changes, and rising biomarkers, as well as any patient with hemodynamic or electrical instability. In such cases urgent PCI is advisable, and the choice and timing of adjuvant antiplatelet and anticoagulant therapies are similar to the case of STEMI with primary PCI.

For patients who are stable but have a moderate to high risk score, PCI is generally planned within 24 to 48 hours of admission. Routine up-front administration of a GPIIb/IIIa inhibitor is not generally recommended, due to excess bleeding risk. Unless there is a high suspicion that the patient will require urgent CABG, administration of clopidogrel before PCI is reasonable, and either enoxaparin or heparin may be started in the ED. If the patient becomes unexpectedly more unstable, a GPIIb/IIIa inhibitor can be added as plans are made for urgent PCI.

For patients who are deemed to be at low risk and in whom a noninvasive strategy is planned, clopidogrel should still be administered, and enoxaparin is preferred as an anticoagulant. In patients with an increased risk of bleeding, fondaparinux is an acceptable alternative.

SUMMARY

ACS is a diagnosis that is made daily in the ED and includes a spectrum of disease ranging from STEMI to low-risk NSTE-ACS. The diagnosis of ACS depends variably on a combination of clinical symptoms, ECG findings, and cardiac biomarkers. Management of ACS is targeted at restoring and maintaining coronary blood flow and improving myocardial oxygen balance. The intensity of treatment, ranging from fibrinolytic therapy and primary PCI on the one hand to conservative and supportive therapy on the other, is commensurate with the severity of disease and the opportunity to improve short-term morbidity and mortality.

REFERENCES

1. Rogers VL, Go AS, Lloyd-Jones DM, et al. Heart disease and stroke statistics—2011 update: a report from the American Heart Association. Circulation 2011;123: e18–209.
2. Iribarren C, Go AS, Husson G. Metabolic syndrome and early-onset coronary artery disease: is the whole greater than its parts. J Am Coll Cardiol 2006;48: 1800–7.
3. Berger A, Meier JM, Stauffer JC. ECG interpretation during the acute phase of coronary syndromes: In need of improvement? Swiss Med Wkly 2004;134:695–9.
4. Roe MT, Parsons LS, Pollack CV Jr, et al; for the National Registry of Myocardial Infarction Investigators. Quality of care by classification of myocardial infarction: treatment patterns for ST-segment elevation vs non-ST-segment elevation myocardial infarction. Arch Intern Med 2005;165:1630–6.
5. Ghaemmaghami CA, Burt DR. Acute reperfusion therapy in acute myocardial infarction. Emerg Med Clin North Am 2005;23(4):1043–63.
6. Antman EM, Hand M, Armstrong PW, et al. Focused update of the ACC/AHA 2004 guidelines for the management of patients with ST-elevation myocardial infarction. J Am Coll Cardiol 2008;51:210–47.

7. Slater DK, Hlatky MA, Mark DB, et al. Outcomes in suspected acute myocardial infarction with normal or minimally abnormal admission electrocardiographic findings. Am J Cardiol 1987;60(10):766–70.

8. Thrombolytic Therapy Trialist (FTT) Collaborative Group. Indications for thrombolytic therapy in suspected acute myocardial infarction: collaborative overview of early mortality and major morbidity results from all randomized trial of more than 1000 patients. Lancet 1994;343:311–22.

9. Randomised trial of intravenous streptokinase, oral aspirin, both, or neither among 17,187 cases of suspected acute myocardial infarction: ISIS-2. Lancet 1988;2(8607):349–60.

10. Maalouf R, Mosley M, James KK, et al. A comparison of salicylic acid levels in normal subjects after rectal versus oral dosing. Acad Emerg Med 2009;16(2): 157–61.

11. Harrington RA, Becker RC, Ezekowitz M, et al. Antithrombotic therapy for coronary artery disease: the Seventh ACCP Conference on Antithrombotic and Thrombolytic Therapy. Chest 2004;126(Suppl 3):513S–48S.

12. Antman EM, Anbe DT, Armstrong PW, et al. ACC/AHA guidelines for the management of patients with ST-elevation myocardial infarction: a report of the American College of Cardiology/American Heart Association Task Force on Practice Guidelines (Committee to Revise the 1999 Guidelines for the Management of Patients with Acute Myocardial Infarction). J Am Coll Cardiol 2004;44(3): E1–211.

13. Fourth International study of Infarct survival Collaborative Group (ISIS-4). A randomized factorial trial assessing early oral captopril, oral mononitrate, and intravenous magnesium sulphate in 58,050 patients with suspected acute myocardial infarction. Lancet 1995;345(8951):669–85.

14. Rude RE, Muller JE, Braunwald E. Effort to limit the size of myocardial infarcts. Ann Intern Med 1981;95(6):735–61.

15. Meine TJ, Roe MT, Chen AY, et al. Association of intravenous morphine use and outcomes in acute coronary syndromes: results from the CRUSADE Quality Improvement Initiative. Am Heart J 2005;149(6):1043–9.

16. Roberts R, Rogers WF, Mueller HS, et al. Immediate versus deferred beta-blockade following thrombolytic therapy in patients with acute myocardial infarction. Results of the Thrombolysis in Myocardial Infarction (TIMI) II-B Study. Circulation 1991; 83(2):422–37.

17. Chen ZM, Pan HC, Chen YP, et al; COMMIT (ClOpidogrel and Metoprolol in Myocardial Infarction Trial) collaborative group. Early intravenous then oral metoprolol in 45,852 patients with acute myocardial infarction: randomised placebo-controlled trial. Lancet 2005;366(9497):1622–32.

18. Antman EM, Hand M, Armstrong PW, et al. 2007 focused update of the ACC/AHA 2004 guidelines for the management of patients with ST-elevation myocardial infarction: a report of the American College of Cardiology/American Heart Association Task Force on Practice Guidelines. Circulation 2008;117(2): 296–329.

19. Assessment of the Safety and Efficacy of a New Treatment Strategy with Percutaneous Coronary Intervention (SENT-4 PCI) Investigators. Primary versus tenecteplase facilitated percutaneous coronary intervention in patient with ST-segment elevation myocardial infarction. Lancet 2006;367(9510):569–78.

20. Keeley EC, Bonura JA, Grines CL. Primary angioplasty versus intravenous thrombolytic therapy for acute myocardial infarction: a quantitative review of 23 randomised trials. Lancet 2003;361(9351):13–20.

21. Boersman E, Primary Coronary Angioplasty vs Thrombolysis Group. Does time matter? A pooled analysis of randomized clinical trials comparing primary percutaneous coronary intervention and in-hospital fibrinolysis in acute myocardial infarction patients. Eur Heart J 2006;27(7):779–88.

22. Ellis SG, Tendera M, de Belder MA, et al. Facilitated PCI in patients with ST-elevation myocardial infarction. N Engl J Med 2008;358(21):2205–17.

23. McKay RG, Dada MR, Mather JF, et al. Comparison of outcomes and safety of "facilitated" versus primary percutaneous coronary intervention in patients with ST-Segment myocardial infarction. Am J Cardiol 2009;103(3):316–21.

24. Keeley EC, Boura JA, Grines CL. Comparison of primary and facilitated percutaneous coronary interventions for ST-elevation myocardial infarction: quantitative review of randomized trials. Lancet 2006;367(9510):579–88.

25. Donnan GA, Fisher M, Macleod M, et al. Stroke. Lancet 2008;371(9624):1612–23.

26. Hochman JS, Lamas GA, Butler CE, et al. Coronary intervention for persistent occlusion after myocardial infarction. N Engl J Med 2006;355:2395–407.

27. Ryan TJ, Anderson JL, Antman EM, et al. ACC/AHA guidelines for the management of patients with acute myocardial infarction. A report of the American College of Cardiology/American Heart Association Task Force on Practice Guidelines. J Am Coll Cardiol 1996;28(5):1328–428.

28. RxList: Internet Drug Index. Available at: http://www.rxlist.com/script/main/hp.asp. Accessed September 2, 2011.

29. Pharmacy Healthcare Solutions. Thrombolytics: therapeutic class review. Eden Prairie (MN): Amerisource Bergen; 2003. p. 7. Available at: http://www.pharmhs.com/Forms/Thrombolytics%20Review.pdf. Accessed September 2, 2011.

30. Merck manuals online medical library for healthcare professionals. IV fibrinolytic drugs available in the US. Available at: http://www.merck.com/media/mmpe/pdf/Table_073-7.pdf. Accessed September 2, 2011.

31. Tarascon pocket pharmacopoeia: 2010 classic shirt-pocket edition. Lompoco (CA): Tarascon Publishing; 2008.

32. Brady W, Harrington RA, Chan T. Section III: acute coronary syndromes. In: Marx A, Hickberger RS, Walls RM, editors. Rosen's emergency medicine: concepts and clinical practice. Part 3. 6th edition. St Louis (MO): CV Mosby; 2006. p. 1165–9.

33. Stone GW, McLaurin BT, Cox DA, et al. Bivalrudin for patient with acute coronary syndrome. N Engl J Med 2006;355(21):2203–16.

A Phased Approach to Cardiac Arrest Resuscitation Involving Ventricular Fibrillation and Pulseless Ventricular Tachycardia

John P. Benner, BA, NREMT-P[a,b], Sarah Morris, MD[c],
William J. Brady, MD[a,c,d],*

KEYWORDS

• Cardiac arrest • Resuscitation • Ventricular fibrillation
• Ventricular tachycardia

The management of out-of-hospital cardiac arrest (OHCA) has undergone significant change over the past decade.[1] Traditional—and outdated—approaches[2] to OHCA resuscitation were complex, with heavy emphasis on early advanced life support (ALS) interventions. American Heart Association (AHA) Guidelines prior to 2000 featured invasive airway management, oxygenation/ventilation by bag-valve mask (BVM), cardiopulmonary resuscitation (CPR), and other procedure-based therapies, all as top priorities in the initial stages of resuscitation, with the assumption that high-quality CPR was performed. Following the release of the AHA Guidelines 2000 and 2005, the focus was on basic life support (BLS), with greater emphasis on early defibrillation of ventricular fibrillation (VF),[3] increasing the quality of chest compressions, and a smaller ventilation-to-chest compression ratio.[4] Today, with the recent release of the 2010 AHA Guidelines for CPR and emergency cardiac care (ECC), the evidence suggests an even more fundamental approach. While the guidelines include many important changes, by far the most notable is the replacement of the long

[a] Charlottesville-Albemarle Rescue Squad, Charlottesville, VA 22901, USA
[b] Virginia College of Osteopathic Medicine, Blacksburg, VA 24060, USA
[c] Department of Emergency Medicine, University of Virginia School of Medicine, Charlottesville, VA 22908, USA
[d] Albemarle County Fire Rescue, Charlottesville, VA 22901, USA
* Corresponding author. Department of Emergency Medicine, University of Virginia School of Medicine, Charlottesville, VA 22908.
E-mail address: wb4z@virginia.edu

Emerg Med Clin N Am 29 (2011) 711–719
doi:10.1016/j.emc.2011.08.003
0733-8627/11/$ – see front matter © 2011 Elsevier Inc. All rights reserved.

emed.theclinics.com

traditional "ABCs" (Airway, Breathing, Circulation) with the "CABs" (Chest compressions, Airway, Breathing), forcing a necessary emphasis on compressions. To aid in understanding and learning, the authors propose a method that optimizes the timing and delivery of evidence-proven therapies with a 3-phase approach for out-of-hospital resuscitation from VF and pulseless ventricular tachycardia (VT). Although this model is not a new concept,[2,3,5] it is largely based on the 2010 AHA Guidelines, enhancing the philosophy of the CABs.

THE EVIDENCE

The wealth of research in support of the 2010 AHA Guidelines is tremendous. Many of these investigations demonstrate that increased survival can be achieved by reorganizing the execution of care provided at the bystander and emergency medical services (EMS) level, specifically in the areas of CPR, early defibrillation, oxygenation, ventilation, and airway management. Because much of this research is also the foundation for the authors' proposed phased approach to VF/pulseless VT resuscitation, the crucial research is discussed here, followed by a discussion of the phased approach.

Chest Compressions and Rescue Breathing

One of the key components of the 2010 AHA Guidelines[1] is the change from performing the ABCs to performing the CABs,[6] demonstrating how important compressions are relative to airway management and oxygenation, particularly at the early stage of a cardiac arrest. Recently, chest-compression-only CPR, without mouth-to-mouth breathing, variously known as "hands only" CPR (HOCPR), cardiocerebral resuscitation, continuous chest compression, or minimally interrupted CPR, has been proposed as an alternative method of resuscitation after cardiac arrest. As noted, rescue breathing is of limited benefit in cardiac arrest, because of pulseless VT and VF in the early phase of management. HOCPR has been shown to have similar efficacy to conventional CPR with the outcome of neurologically intact survival 1 year after a witnessed arrest of presumed cardiac origin.[7] In patients with an initially shockable rhythm, Kellum and colleagues[8] demonstrated an increased survival rate with neurologically intact status after receiving HOCPR. In 2000, a somewhat larger trial of OHCA patients who received HOCPR as compared with conventional CPR showed equal survival to hospital discharge as well as an equal number of patients alive, with no morbidity at 2.4 years after their event; in fact, survival was noted in 35 of 240 (15%) of HOCPR recipients versus 29 of 278 (10%) treated with conventional CPR.[9]

Additional evidence is found in the SOS-KANTO (Survey of Survivors after out-of hospital cardiac arrest in the Kanto area of Japan) trial; this study reviewed 4068 witnessed OHCAs, of which 1151 patients received bystander CPR. The 439 subjects who received HOCPR showed similar neurologic outcome at 30 days in comparison with conventional CPR (6% vs 4% of survivors). There was no benefit seen with the addition of mouth-to-mouth ventilation.[10] It should be noted that there were significant differences in the study groups, including more males and more arrests at home in the HOCPR group. Furthermore, in 2008 Bobrow and colleagues[11] demonstrated that cycles of 200 continuous compressions, followed by an electrical defibrillation with immediate resumption of compressions before endotracheal intubation, resulted in increased survival (1.8% vs 5.4%) in all patients; in the witnessed VF subgroup, survival increased from 4.7% to 17.6%.

Reasons for this change from ABCs to the CABs are many, but several investigators point out that continuous chest compressions are not always performed as taught in the classroom.[12,13] In fact, chest compressions are often delayed, frequently interrupted, and of poor quality. In a study of OHCAs, Wik and colleagues[14] found that CPR was only performed 48% of the time when indicated, and when it was performed the mean rate was only 64 compressions per minute, reaching an appropriate depth (at least 5 cm) in only 28% of the cases. In a similar in-hospital cardiac arrest study, Abella and colleagues[15,16] found that nearly 40% of resuscitations included suboptimal CPR, performed at rates below 80 compressions per minute. Wang and colleagues[17] reported that CPR was frequently interrupted for prolonged periods, anywhere from 1.8 to 7 minutes, to perform endotracheal intubation.[18] Similarly, Valenzuela and colleagues[3] found two major problems in their study of OHCAs regarding interruptions during CPR: (1) EMS providers were only performing CPR 40% $\pm$ 21% of the time within the first 5 minutes of patient care, and (2) multiple factors substantially delayed CPR, including extraneous reassessments of pulse, placing intravenous lines, and the performance of intubation with frequent reassessment of tube placement. Finally, Aufderheide and colleagues[12] observed that adult, intubated OHCA patients were hyperventilated during CPR at an average rate of 30 $\pm$ 2 breaths per minute, when the suggested rate is approximately 8 to 10 per minute. These groups correlate poor quality and interrupted CPR with increased mortality, decreased rate of return of spontaneous circulation (ROSC), and poor rates of survival that occurred in each of their studies.

Recognizing the physiology behind CPR, specifically relating to chest compressions, is critical to its application in the field. It has been postulated that a victim of sudden, unexpected VF collapses with his or her lungs, pulmonary veins, left heart, and entire arterial system full of oxygen,[2] and this amount of oxygenated blood may be sufficient to perfuse vital tissues for a short period,[11] if circulated with CPR promptly following collapse. The level of perfusion pressure provided during uninterrupted CPR is not equivalent to that of a healthy beating heart. In fact, high-quality CPR provides markedly reduced levels of cardiac output, with hemodynamics very similar to cardiogenic shock.[19] However, the small pressures provided by chest compressions can provide a huge impact on survival, but there is no question that they must be performed correctly. At initiation of CPR, it takes time for good compressions to increase coronary and cerebral perfusion pressures to mean threshold levels considered "adequate" for perfusion of vital organs. This theory is analogous to "momentum." Any interruption of compressions causes the blood flow to lose momentum, and the loss of perfusion below threshold levels to each vital organ, only to waste precious time starting all over again at perfusion pressures of 0 mm Hg as CPR is resumed.[2,20,21] There may be some increased benefit to using mechanical CPR devices; although conflicting studies do exist, these devices are able to deliver higher perfusion pressures above threshold in comparison with manual CPR, thus increasing survival in some studies.[22] Whether using manual or mechanical CPR, the physiology remains the same. To maximize the performance of CPR, the following factors must be ensured: chest compressions must be forceful and fast, at rates greater than 100 per minute[6,15]; representing systole, compression depth (at least 5 cm) must be sufficient to deliver adequate stroke volume and cerebral perfusion pressure[4,23]; representing diastole, full chest recoil must be permitted after every compression to allow for filling of the ventricles and coronary perfusion pressure to fill the coronary arteries[2]; during the early phase, CPR must not be interrupted, even for ventilations,[11,19] unless the reason for interruption is more important to survival than perfusing the heart and brain[2,8,24]—the only intervention of this type is early defibrillation, and pauses during CPR both preshock and postshock should be kept as short as possible[13,25]; if ventilations are provided, they must be provided at a compression to ventilation ratio of 30:2[6] and a rate of no greater than 8 to 10 per minute, because hyperventilation in this setting is associated with increased thoracic pressure, decreasing venous return to the heart, and further limiting cardiac output crucial to survival.[2,12] When performed correctly and coupled with early bystander CPR, uninterrupted chest compressions are clearly the most important determinant in achieving neurologically intact survival from OHCA.[2,9–11,19,24,26,27]

Early Defibrillation

Considered one of the only acceptable reasons to interrupt CPR during early VF arrest, prompt defibrillation is critical to survival in this setting. Unquestionably, the best time to defibrillate is when a monitored patient first decompensates to VF or pulseless VT.[11] Similarly, the utility of early defibrillation has been well demonstrated by the nearly twofold increase in survival following early use of public-access automated external defibrillators (AEDs).[19] Considering that most OHCAs do not occur in the presence of a defibrillator, the best time to perform it when the device arrives to the scene of an arrest has been an important question for many investigators. The longer VF continues without conversion to a perfusing rhythm, progressive myocardial substrate (adenosine triphosphate [ATP]) depletion occurs, with wastes accumulating at the same rate. The higher the myocardial ATP stores, the more likely a defibrillation attempt will successfully convert to a perfusing rhythm; however, the more wastes that are present in myocytes, the higher the likelihood of defibrillation failure, converting VF into pulseless electrical activity (PEA) or asystole.[2,11,26] On analysis of VF morphology, course VF signifies that the myocytes are ATP-rich, whereas fine VF indicates potential ATP depletion. Without prompt treatment, coarse VF will degenerate into fine VF, and ultimately asystole.[11,13] When 2 minutes of good-quality CPR is performed before and after defibrillation,[2] wastes are able to be removed from the myocytes and substrates are renewed, increasing the likelihood that defibrillation will convert VF to a perfusing rhythm.

Multiple investigators describe that EMS is more likely to arrive on-scene and start resuscitative efforts around or after the 5-minute mark of a witnessed VF OHCA. Hayakawa and colleagues[26] performed a study on the likelihood of survival based on the influence of CPR before or after defibrillation. Several important observations were made. EMS arrived past the 5-minute mark in 90% of cases. The shock-first group, waiting more than 5 minutes for the first shock, had worse neurologically intact survival than did the CPR-first group (11% vs 26% at 1-year follow-up, respectively). Further, the CPR-first group received a mean of 3.7 ± 2.2 minutes of CPR before defibrillation. Wik and colleagues[28] investigated a mean CPR duration of 3 minutes before defibrillation, with a 20% versus 15% 1-year survival rate for the CPR-first group and the shock-first group, respectively. All of these studies featured a downtime of greater than 5 minutes, and neither of the two groups differed in their ROSC rates, but neurologically intact survival at 1 year was significantly better for the CPR-first groups. Cobb and colleagues[23] found that with 90 seconds of CPR before defibrillation of VF patients down longer than 4 minutes had an increase in survival from 24% to 30%. However, in contrast to all of these studies, neither Baker and colleagues[29] nor Jacobs and colleagues[30] found any correlation of increased survival with CPR first before rapid defibrillation for longer downtimes of VF; both groups support immediate defibrillation no matter the downtime if VF is the presenting rhythm. Despite the latter two findings, performance of CPR before the first defibrillation for downtimes longer than 4 to 5 minutes should be considered because the evidence in favor of any amount of CPR first has been shown to be beneficial.[6,23,26,28] These studies highlight the need for CPR first, interrupted only briefly for single defibrillation attempts, during the middle phase of VF OHCA.

Oxygenation/Ventilation/Airway Management

The provision of ventilations by BVM is controversial because of new theories regarding the potential increase in intrathoracic pressure, decreasing venous return and, therefore, cardiac output.[12] However, the physiology and evidence regarding passive oxygenation with 100% oxygen by non-rebreather (NRB) instead during initial phases of a VF arrest is intriguing, and should be considered when sufficient personnel are not available to operate a BVM, as recommended by the 2010 AHA Guidelines. At this point, there is insufficient evidence to consider removing BVM ventilations in favor of passive ventilations.[6] In accordance with the new guidelines, performance of BVM ventilations and invasive airway placement should be considered, especially during the later phases of resuscitation.

Oxygenation and ventilation do occur to a substantial degree during unventilated chest compressions, secondary to chest compression-induced gas exchange, with small volumes of air exhaled and inhaled on compression and recoil, respectively.[11] In addition, gasping (agonal breathing) is often witnessed during VF arrests, determined not only as a favorable sign for survival,[2,20,27,31] but also as a potential means for oxygen inhalation.[11] Several studies have shown that oxygenation/ventilation may not be as necessary in the first 6 to 12 minutes of a resuscitation, as in later phases of an arrest.[2,7,12,20,21,32] The previously mentioned SOS-KANTO trial studied the benefits of bystander CPR with rescue breaths versus compression-only CPR without ventilations, and found that CPR without ventilations was far superior.[20] Aufderheide and colleagues[12] studied hyperventilation in a swine model, reporting that positive pressure ventilation increased intrathoracic pressure, thereby decreasing venous return, and further decreasing perfusion pressures resulting in decreased ROSC. Given all of these variables, Bobrow and colleagues[32] studied the outcomes of VF initially ventilated passively with 100% FiO_2 by NRB mask versus those ventilated with a BVM. The passive group was then intubated after 3 CPR-defibrillation cycles. The passive ventilation group carried a 38.2% survival to hospital discharge rate, double that of the BVM group. Kellum and colleagues[8] performed an almost identical study, with an astounding result of 47% survival (from 15%), with 39% neurologically intact at hospital discharge. Although the above studies certainly show the effects of providing increased oxygen content to the blood, each considers that the primary power is more in the method of oxygen delivery, by decreasing interruptions during CPR, thereby increasing survival. However, in considering exceptions to this model, Bobrow and colleagues reported no immediate benefit in patients presenting with a nonshockable rhythm, further demonstrating that more research is needed before this method can be extended beyond VF arrests.

Indeed, this massive body of research clearly outlines the critical need for fundamental changes in resuscitation methodology, to which the 2010 AHA Guidelines have responded and thoroughly addressed. With this research and the new guidelines in mind, the authors propose a method that goes one step further: a 3-phase approach to VF and pulseless VT OHCA resuscitation. This approach is not a new concept, with several investigators having proposed similar methods in recent years.[2,3,5] However, this reconceptualized approach includes the new AHA Guidelines and the crucial evidence leading to their creation.

THE PHASES OF RESUSCITATION

Also known as "cardiocerebral resuscitation," the 3-phased approach has been discussed as an effective means of reorganizing delivery of the critical components of resuscitative care.[2,3,5,8,11,27] This method divides the process of OHCA resuscitation into 3 distinct phases, each outlined with rhythm-specific, time-sensitive priorities based on the corresponding pathophysiologic process likely to occur during each period. The goal is to optimize survival by providing the maximally effective initial therapy for each particular phase of an arrest.[5] Each proven therapy should be applied under conditions most favoring an ROSC, as in the setting of a witnessed sudden, cardiac arrest with VF or pulseless VT as the primary or presenting rhythm. The initial rhythm and likely etiology are the key elements in using this resuscitation model. Whereas VF is widely known as a survivable rhythm in the setting of prompt defibrillation,[25] PEA and asystole are associated with multiple complex illnesses causing cardiac arrest, and often lead to poor outcomes.[5] Similarly, certain types of arrests, like those with respiratory components (eg, exacerbation of chronic obstructive pulmonary disease) or hypovolemia (eg, septic shock) have not been proved to respond favorably to the phased approach.[2,3,5,11,26,27,33]

The Early Phase

The OHCA begins in the "Early" phase, encompassing approximately the first 5 to 8 minutes in patients with VF or pulseless VT. Termed by investigators the "electrical" phase,[2,3,5,27,33] early defibrillation is the best intervention during this period, accompanied by maintenance of coronary and cerebral perfusion pressure through continuous, high-quality chest compressions.[2,5,15,34] On arrival of EMS or an AED, if the patient's downtime is less than 4 to 5 minutes an immediate single defibrillation should be considered; for downtimes exceeding that time frame, chest compressions should be performed for 2 minutes and then a single defibrillation considered.[6,23,28,32] The evidence supporting this statement is mixed, however, such that the AHA now states that health care providers must determine the most appropriate time for defibrillation based on patient needs and system abilities.[1]

Passive insufflation of oxygen should be initially considered by NRB mask at 100% FiO_2 during CPR if the airway is patent,[32] or by BVM if at least 2 personnel are present. However, neither oxygenation nor ventilation have proven to be necessary in the first few minutes of a VF arrest; this changes as the arrest moves into the Middle phase, when they become essential.[7,10,20] Interrupting and delaying chest compressions for endotracheal intubation (ETI) during this phase is not recommended,[2,17,18] and should only be considered for Early-phase rhythm or illness exceptions (see below). Intravenous/intraosseous access and standard vasopressor and antiarrhythmic medications should be administered by local protocol, but this intervention should not interrupt chest compressions.

Recognition of Early-phase exceptions is of utmost importance when using this model of resuscitation. Presenting rhythms, such as PEA and asystole or potential arrest etiology judged to be "noncardiac" or traumatic in nature, should be handled according to the 2010 AHA Advanced Cardiac Life Support (ACLS) guidelines for each specific presentation. If the arrest is caused primarily by a respiratory illness, early invasive airway placement and aggressive oxygenation during the Early and Middle phases is indicated; similarly, hypovolemic states require intravenous volume replacement and medication therapy during all 3 phases.[3,5,7,8,27,31,33,35] Nonetheless, in these "exception scenarios," high-quality chest compressions are still vital to successful resuscitation outcome.

The Middle Phase

Phase 2, the "Middle" phase, spans approximately the next 5 minutes, and is known as the "circulatory or hemodynamic" phase.[2,3,5,27,33] Here, maintenance of coronary and cerebral perfusion pressures is critical to neurologically intact survival, more so than is defibrillation.[2] Oxygenation and ventilation by bag-mask technique should be provided at this point in the arrest. An immediate defibrillation can be considered if bystander CPR is being performed on arrival of EMS; in all other cases, however, chest compressions should be performed for at least 2 minutes before and after the first defibrillation attempt. Because the evidence does show that Middle-phase defibrillations need to interrupt CPR, these interruption durations should be minimized. Shallow chest compressions and long preshock and postshock pauses of CPR should be avoided, as they have been associated with defibrillation failure and decreased ROSC.[10,13,26,28] Securing the airway by invasive means is the second priority of this phase, and should be attempted after 3 chest compression-defibrillation cycles. If 2 providers are present, BVM ventilations should be considered. If ETI is successful, end-tidal CO_2 monitoring should be performed.[6,17]

The Late Phase

The "Late" phase comprises the remainder of the resuscitation and is termed the "metabolic" phase.[2,3,5,27,33] Initiating or maintaining standard ACLS interventions and medications is the goal for this phase, as the pure physiologic benefits of early defibrillation and chest compressions that comprise the Early and Middle phases are less likely to contribute to ROSC this late in the resuscitation.[2,3,5,27,33] However, each should still be performed as needed until ROSC is achieved or the resuscitation is terminated.

Novel interventions not discussed in this article include the induction of hypothermia[36,37] and the use of an impedance threshold device.[35,38] Both have been shown to improve survival, and depending on the timing of their application, each may contribute significantly to any one of these phases of resuscitation.

SUMMARY

This proposed approach is meant to organize the time-critical components into phases for the care of the witnessed, VF OHCA patient, providing a basic framework based on the most up-to-date resuscitation evidence available. Current recommendations for detailed information, such as actual phase durations, durations of therapies and procedures, novel interventions, drugs and dosages used, postresuscitative care, and so forth, should be based not on this article, but on medical director–determined local protocols and the 2010 AHA Guidelines for CPR and ECC. The key components are early defibrillation of VF, minimizing interruptions of CPR (to no interruptions, if possible), and early identification of illness or rhythm-based exceptions to this model.

REFERENCES

1. Field JM, Hazinski MF, Sayre MR, et al. 2010 American Heart Association guidelines for cardiopulmonary resuscitation and emergency cardiovascular care science. Circulation 2010;122:S640–946.
2. Ewy GA. Cardiocerebral resuscitation: the new cardiopulmonary resuscitation. Circulation 2005;111:2134–42.
3. Valenzuela TD, Kern KB, Clark LL, et al. Interruptions of chest compressions during emergency medical systems resuscitation. Circulation 2005;112:1259–65.
4. ECC Committee, Subcommittees and Task Forces of the American Heart Association. 2005 American Heart Association guidelines for cardiopulmonary resuscitation and emergency cardiovascular care. Circulation 2005;112(Suppl 24): IV1–203.

5. Weisfeldt ML, Becker LB. Resuscitation after cardiac arrest: a 3-phase time-sensitive model. JAMA 2002;288(23):3035–8.

6. Neumar RW, Otto CW, Link MS, et al. 2010 AHA guidelines for CPR and ECC, part 8: adult advanced cardiovascular life support. Circulation 2010;122(Suppl 3): S729–67.

7. Iwami T, Kawamura T, Hiraide A, et al. Effectiveness of bystander-initiated cardiac-only resuscitation for patients with out-of-hospital cardiac arrest. Circulation 2007;116:2900–7.

8. Kellum MJ, Kennedy KW, Barney R, et al. Cardiocerebral resuscitation improves neurologically intact survival of patients with out-of-hospital cardiac arrest. Ann Emerg Med 2008;52:244–52.

9. Hallstrom A, Cobb L, Johnson E, et al. Cardiopulmonary resuscitation by chest compression alone or with mouth-to-mouth ventilation. N Engl J Med 2000; 342(21):1546–53.

10. Ewy GA. Continuous-chest-compression cardiopulmonary resuscitation for cardiac arrest. Circulation 2007;116:2894–6.

11. Bobrow BJ, Clark LL, Ewy GA, et al. Minimally interrupted cardiac resuscitation by emergency medical services for out-of-hospital cardiac arrest. JAMA 2008; 299(10):1158–65.

12. Aufderheide TP, Sigurdsson G, Pirrallo RG, et al. Hyperventilation-induced hypotension during cardiopulmonary resuscitation. Circulation 2004;109:1960–5.

13. Edelson DP, Abella BS, Kramer-Johansen J, et al. Effects of compression depth and pre-shock pauses predict defibrillation failure during cardiac arrest. Resuscitation 2006;71:137–45.

14. Wik L, Kramer-Johansen J, Myklebust H, et al. Quality of cardiopulmonary resuscitation during out-of-hospital cardiac arrest. JAMA 2005;293(3):299–304.

15. Abella BS, Sandbo N, Vassilatos P, et al. Chest compression rates during cardiopulmonary resuscitation are suboptimal: a prospective study during in-hospital cardiac arrest. Circulation 2005;111:428–34.

16. Abella BS, Alvarado JP, Myklebust H, et al. Quality of cardiopulmonary resuscitation during in-hospital cardiac arrest. JAMA 2005;293(3):305–10.

17. Wang HE, Simeone SJ, Weaver MD, et al. Interruptions in cardiopulmonary resuscitation from paramedic endotracheal intubation. Ann Emerg Med 2009;54:645–52.

18. Bobrow BJ, Spaite DW. Do not pardon the interruption. Ann Emerg Med 2009;54: 653–5.

19. Weisfeldt ML, Ornato JP. Closed-chest cardiac massage: progress measured by the exceptions. JAMA 2008;300(13):1582–4.

20. SOS-KANTO study group. Cardiopulmonary resuscitation by bystanders with chest compression only (SOS-KANTO): an observational study. Lancet 2007;369:920–6.

21. Berg RA, Sanders AB, Kern KB, et al. Adverse hemodynamic effects of interrupting chest compressions for rescue breathing during cardiopulmonary resuscitation for ventricular fibrillation cardiac arrest. Circulation 2001;104:2465–70.

22. Hallstrom A, Rea TD, Sayre MR, et al. Manual chest compression vs use of an automated chest compression device during resuscitation following out-of-hospital cardiac arrest: a randomized trial. JAMA 2006;295:2620–8.

23. Cobb LA, Fahrenbruch CE, Walsh TR, et al. Influence of cardiopulmonary resuscitation prior to defibrillation in patients with out-of-hospital ventricular fibrillation. JAMA 1999;281(13):1182–8.

24. Kern KB, Hilwig RW, Berg RA, et al. Importance of continuous chest compressions during cardiopulmonary resuscitation: improved outcome during a simulated single lay-rescuer scenario. Circulation 2002;105:645–9.

25. Sell RE, Sarno R, Lawrence B. Minimizing pre- and post-defibrillation pauses increases the likelihood of return of spontaneous circulation (ROSC). Resuscitation 2010;81:822–5.
26. Hayakawa M, Gando S, Okamoto H, et al. Shortening of cardiopulmonary resuscitation time before the defibrillation worsens the outcome in out-of-hospital VF patients. Am J Emerg Med 2009;27:470–4.
27. Bobrow BJ, Ewy GA. Ventilation during resuscitation efforts for out-of-hospital primary cardiac arrest. Curr Opin Crit Care 2009;15:228–33.
28. Wik L, Hansen TB, Fylling F, et al. Delaying defibrillation to give basic cardiopulmonary resuscitation to patients with out-of-hospital ventricular fibrillation: a randomized trial. JAMA 2003;289(11):1389–95.
29. Baker PW, Conway J, Cotton C, et al. Defibrillation or cardiopulmonary resuscitation first for patients with out-of-hospital cardiac arrests found by paramedics to be in ventricular fibrillation? A randomised control trial. Resuscitation 2008;79: 424–31.
30. Jacobs IG, Finn JC, Oxer HF, et al. CPR before defibrillation in out-of-hospital cardiac arrest: a randomized trial. Emerg Med Australas 2005;17:39–45.
31. Seethala RR, Abella BS. To ventilate or not to ventilate during cardiopulmonary resuscitation: that is the question. Heart 2010;96:577–8.
32. Bobrow BJ, Ewy GA, Clark L, et al. Passive oxygen insufflation is superior to bag-valve-mask ventilation for witnessed ventricular fibrillation out-of-hospital cardiac arrest. Ann Emerg Med 2009;54:656–62.
33. Sanders AB. Progress in improving neurologically intact survival from cardiac arrest. Ann Emerg Med 2008;52:253–5.
34. Sayre MR, Berg RA, Cave DM, et al. Hands-only (compression-only) cardiopulmonary resuscitation: a call to action for bystander response to adults who experience out-of-hospital sudden cardiac arrest: a science advisory for the public from the American Heart Association Emergency Cardiovascular Care Committee. Circulation 2008;117:2162–7.
35. Aufderheide TP, Alexander C, Lick C, et al. From laboratory science to six emergency medical services systems: new understanding of the physiology of cardiopulmonary resuscitation increases survival rates after cardiac arrest. Crit Care Med 2008;36(Suppl):S397–404.
36. Vanden Hoek TL, Kasza KE, Beiser DG, et al. Induced hypothermia by central venous infusion: saline ice slurry versus chilled saline. Crit Care Med 2004; 32(9):S425–31.
37. Hinchey PR, Myers JB, Lewis R, et al. Improved out-of-hospital cardiac arrest survival after the sequential implementation of 2005 AHA guidelines for compressions, ventilations, and induced hypothermia; the Wake County experience. Ann Emerg Med 2010;56:348–57.
38. Cabrini L, Beccaria P, Landoni G, et al. Impact of impedance threshold devices on cardiopulmonary resuscitation: a systematic review and meta-analysis of randomized controlled studies. Crit Care Med 2008;36(5):1625–32.

Approach to the ED Patient with "Low-Risk" Chest Pain

Joshua M. Kosowsky, MD

KEYWORDS

• Chest pain • Low risk • Emergency department

There is abundant evidence to guide the management of patients with chest pain with a confirmed or reasonably suspected diagnosis of acute coronary syndrome (ACS), but when it comes to the patient with "low-risk chest pain" in the emergency department (ED), there is limited evidence to support one approach over another. As a result, the evaluation of low-risk chest pain represents a distinct challenge for the emergency physician. Missing a diagnosis of ACS is, of course, undesirable. At the same time, the overuse of technology can result in misleading test results in populations with a low incidence of coronary disease.

For emergency physicians in most developed countries, chest pain is a high-frequency, high-risk, chief complaint. US statistics show that in 2007, there were approximately 5 million visits to the ED for chest pain.[1] Although more often than not the cause of chest pain turns out to be benign, emergency physicians cannot dismiss the possibility of a life-threatening condition, such as ACS. Historically, anywhere from 2% to 4% of cases of acute myocardial infarction (MI) are missed on initial presentation to the ED. Missing the diagnosis of MI continues to be an area of high medico-legal risk in emergency medicine, accounting for nearly 20% of closed malpractice claims.[2,3] More important, it is of clinical significance that patients who are discharged with a missed diagnosis of MI have a 30-day mortality risk 2 times greater than those who are hospitalized.[2] Acknowledging that not all patients with chest pain can be referred immediately to a cardiologist or admitted to the hospital, emergency physicians have developed strategies for stratifying patients into various risk groups.

The term "low-risk chest pain" does not mean the same thing to everyone. Risk stratification is, by definition, relative to the outcome of concern. Outcomes referenced in the cardiology literature include a diagnosis of MI during a particular clinical encounter, the need for urgent coronary revascularization, the presence of coronary

Department of Emergency Medicine, Brigham and Women's Hospital, 10 Vining Street, Boston, MA 02115, USA
E-mail address: jmkosowsky@partners.org

Emerg Med Clin N Am 29 (2011) 721–727
doi:10.1016/j.emc.2011.09.017
0733-8627/11/$ – see front matter © 2011 Elsevier Inc. All rights reserved.

artery disease (CAD), an eventual diagnosis of cardiac ischemic disease, death from MI, and general mortality. Depending on the setting, these are all valid outcome measures, but for a patient arriving in the ED, the risk of most immediate concern is whether the presenting symptoms are manifestations of ACS, or what may be termed the "incident risk" of ACS.

The incident risk for a particular ED visit is determined from a combination of a patient's demographic risk and the clinical presentation. Generally speaking, a patient's demographic risk has to do with the likelihood that the most common substrate for ACS, namely, CAD, is present. For an individual patient, the likelihood of CAD can be assessed by the traditional risk factors uncovered by the Framingham Study, which include having a first-degree relative with a history of early-life MI, male sex, advanced age, hypertension, smoking history, diabetes, hyperlipidemia, and a family history of early CAD.[4,5] However, although the Framingham score may be useful for predicting future lifetime risk of CAD-related outcomes, studies have shown that a new complaint of chest pain puts that individual at higher short-term risk than any of these historical factors. For example, in men, a family history of early CAD and diabetes increased the relative risk of ACS, but only slightly in comparison with a chief complaint of chest pain and electrocardiogram (ECG) changes.[6] Thus, an over-emphasis on demographic risk to the exclusion of the clinical presentation may result in either undertesting or overtesting.

Although specific definitions of risk categories vary widely, it is generally accepted that patients at "low risk" for ACS can be adequately managed without the need for inpatient hospitalization or the direct involvement of a cardiologist. Over the past 2 decades, the advent of accurate biomarkers for myocardial injury, such as creatine kinase MB fraction (CKMB) and troponin, have allowed for the development of protocols to "rule out" MI within a relatively short period. At the same time, a range of provocative tests, from exercise treadmill testing and stress echocardiography to nuclear imaging studies, are being made available from the ED at many institutions. Emergency physicians are beginning to adopt the practice of using these tests to risk-stratifying patients on the basis of the presence or absence of inducible myocardial ischemia. Most recently, the advent of high-resolution coronary computed tomography angiography (CCTA) allows us to evaluate a patient's coronary anatomy with an accuracy rivaling that of cardiac catheterization. How to integrate these technologies into clinical practice continues to be the subject of considerable debate in the emergency medicine community. In particular, the appeal of high-tech diagnostics must be counterbalanced by the acknowledgment that most of the time, the vast majority of "low-risk" chest pain patients will do well regardless of which strategy is adopted.

CLINICAL HISTORY

Decades of literature have showed that although no one element of the history is sufficiently sensitive or specific to rule in or rule out ACS, there are associations between the quality of chest pain symptoms and the likelihood of ACS. Typical symptoms of ACS include pressurelike chest discomfort; radiation to the arms, neck or shoulders; and associated shortness of breath, diaphoresis, nausea, or anxiety.[7,8] Less typical symptoms include chest pain that is sharp, stabbing, or influenced by position or inspiration. Although less commonly associated with ACS, as many as 1 in 20 patients ultimately diagnosed with acute MI will present with atypical features.[9–11]

There are several recent studies highlighting the limited value of presenting symptoms for making the diagnosis of ACS[12]; however, such studies reduce a patient's narrative to a checklist of items, falling well short of what the experienced clinician garners from even the most cursory history. In fact, a physician's overall clinical gestalt turns out to be one of the best predictors for ACS. A good history remains the cornerstone of diagnosis and, along with the ECG, should serve as a guide to any further diagnostic workup.

ELECTROCARDIOGRAM

Virtually all patients who present to an ED with chest pain will have an ECG performed as part of their initial evaluation. In response to guideline-recommended door-to-ECG times of 10 minutes for patients with ST elevation MI (STEMI), most institutions have developed protocols for patients with chest pain or any ischemic equivalent to receive a screening ECG at or around the time of triage. It must be appreciated, however, that a single ECG represents only a snapshot in what may be a dynamic process in the case of ACS. In patients with hyperacute symptoms, initial ECG findings may be subtle or nonexistent; the hallmark of ACS is that ECG changes tend to evolve over a period of minutes to hours.[13,14] In fact, even among patients who ultimately rule in for MI, an initial "diagnostic" ECG is more the exception than the rule.[15] For this reason, the American College of Emergency Physicians (ACEP) Clinical Policy Committee recommends that for patients with suspected ACS, the ECG be repeated at an interval of 30 to 60 minutes.[16]

CARDIAC BIOMARKERS

Cardiac biomarkers, although variable in their sensitivity and specificity for ACS, remain an important diagnostic tool for the evaluation of the patient with "low-risk" chest pain. In the first few hours after symptom onset, myoglobin has the highest sensitivity of all traditional biomarkers, but with low specificity. After 6 hours, CKMB and troponins have the same sensitivity but with far higher specificity than myoglobin. Earlier generations of troponins and CKMB assays achieve near 100% sensitivity at 12 hours.[17–20] Newer generation troponin I and T assays have demonstrated superior sensitivity, approaching a 94% to 96% at 2 to 4 hours, with 97% to 99% negative predictive value.[21] This makes detection of acute MI possible earlier than ever before.

On the other hand, several caveats are in order. Just as with the ECG, one must take into account the timing of symptoms relative to biomarker measurements. For the patient with chest pain who has been constant for hours or days, it may make abundant sense to rely on a single measurement at or near the time of presentation. On the other hand, for patients whose symptoms are intermittent, the biomarker stopwatch would need to be reset, so to speak, with every recurrence of chest pain. Similarly, if symptom duration is so brief (eg, less than 15–20 minutes) that no significant myocardial injury results, no number of biomarker measurements will be suffice to rule out the possibility of ACS. In that sense, unstable angina remains a clinical diagnosis, although it should be acknowledged that the absence of biomarker positivity portends lower risk (**Fig. 1**).

On the other side of the coin, it needs to be recognized that not all positive troponins represent ACS. Leaving aside the issue of truly "false positive" results (which are exceedingly rare), it has become increasingly clear that not all myocardial damage detected by highly sensitive biomarkers is in fact caused by ACS. In fact, in a typical ED population, elevated troponin levels may be more commonly associated with non-ACS diagnoses (such as congestive heart failure, renal failure, and sepsis) than ACS itself.[22] That said, patients with an elevated troponin, regardless of diagnosis, have higher in-hospital mortality rates and therefore cannot be considered "low risk" in any real sense.[23]

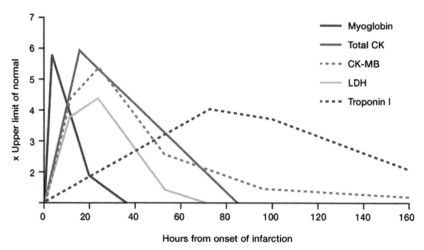

Fig. 1. Myocardial infarction biomarker kinetics.

ADDITIONAL TESTING

For patients with "low-risk" chest pain with no evidence of ongoing myocardial ischemia or infarction after serial ECGs and biomarkers, provocative testing is often used to assess for "inducible" ischemia. EDs that have "chest pain units" or ED observation units are able to achieve nearly 100% compliance with stress testing of patients with "low-risk" chest pain.[24–25] Although American College of Cardiology/American Heart Association guidelines recommend that such patients "may be considered for an early stress test to provoke ischemia … [and] to assess for obstructive CAD,"[26] there is no randomized-trial evidence to support this as universal practice. For one thing, once a patient has "ruled out" for MI with serial biomarkers, the likelihood of an important ACS-related outcome (eg, STEMI, cardiac death) is exceedingly low, so that further risk stratification is inherently difficult. Furthermore, in those studies that have managed to stratify these already "low-risk" patients on the basis of provocative testing, the vast majority of ACS-related outcomes come in the form "urgent revascularization," begging the question of whether those procedures do not simply represent the natural history of a positive or nondiagnostic stress test in the modern era of interventional cardiology. At the end of the day, stress testing in patients with "low-risk" chest pain is relatively low yield in terms of altering subsequent management.[27,28] It is certainly the case that patients who have negative results from the ED can be safely discharged home[29–31]; however, the same is true for patients who are discharged home without additional testing, but with reasonable outpatient follow-up.[32]

Exercise treadmill testing (ETT) is the most commonly used provocative test, and its utility has been tested in a variety of cardiovascular disease populations, most notably as a means of stratifying patients following MI. Overall, the sensitivity (68%) and specificity (77%) of ETT for CAD is limited, with even lower performance in women. For patients with certain baseline ECG abnormalities, utility is rather limited. In an ED population of patients with low-risk chest pain, ETT results have been correlated with cardiovascular outcomes, but absolute rates of coronary events are low in this population regardless. As such, stress testing is prognostic only in those patients with a high pretest probability of CAD.[32]

Although operator dependent, the reported sensitivity and specificity of *stress echocardiography* (Stress Echo) for CAD are than standard ETT.[33,34] As with other imaging techniques, the presence of inducible wall-motion abnormalities are highly sensitive for significant CAD. Additionally, echocardiography provides information on valvular function and contractile performance that may be useful in certain clinical circumstances. Disadvantages of Stress Echo include operator dependence and technical limitations owing to body habitus.

Radionuclide myocardial perfusion imaging (rMPI) involves the use of an injectable radioisotope (such as thallium or sestamibi) to image myocardial perfusion both at rest and with exercise or following a chemically induced ischemic challenge (eg, dipyridamole, persantine, or adenosine). rMPI is generally more expensive and more time-consuming than Stress Echo, and the procedure entails a modest radiation exposure. The results are less operator dependent, however, and when combined with single-photon emission computed tomography (SPECT) imaging, the sensitivity for significant coronary stenosis approaches 90%.

Over the past decade, it has been demonstrated that high-resolution *coronary CT angiography* (CCTA) can approach traditional angiography in defining coronary anatomy. For example, Hoffman and colleagues[35] found that CCTA can identify the presence of and extent of CAD in 80% to 94% of patients. In practice, technical limitations can degrade CCTA image quality, and radiation exposure is a legitimate concern in younger patents. Most important, however, standard CCTA provides no information about myocardial perfusion per se. In other words, although the absence of significant CAD makes ACS extremely unlikely, the presence of CAD does not imply that the patient's chest pain was cardiac in origin.

SUMMARY

Patients who present to the ED with chest pain (or its equivalent) but have no electrocardiographic changes or elevation in cardiac biomarkers after an appropriate interval can be considered low risk for ACS. Combined with a low demographic risk for CAD (eg, using Framingham criteria), such patients can be said to be "low risk" for a subsequent coronary event. Whether there is a role for further risk stratification with provocative testing and/or coronary imaging before discharge remains open to debate.

REFERENCES

1. Bhuiya FA, Pittts SR, McCaig LF. Emergency department visits for chest pain and abdominal pain: United States, 1999–2008. Centers for Disease Control and Prevention. NCHS Data Brief 2010;16(43):1–8.
2. Pope JH, Aufderheide TP, Ruthazer R, et al. Missed diagnosis of acute cardiac ischemia in the emergency department. N Engl J Med 2000;342:1163–70.
3. Mehta RH, Eagle KA. Missed diagnosis of acute coronary syndrome in the emergency room—continuing challenges. N Engl J Med 2000;342(16):1207–9.
4. Gordon T, Sorlie P, Kannel W. Coronary heart disease, atherothrombotic brain infarction, intermittent claudication—a multivariate analysis of some factors related to their incidence: Framingham Study, 16 years follow up. Washington, DC: US Government Printing Office; 1971.
5. Truett J, Cornfield J, Kanell W. A multivariate analysis of the risk of coronary artery disease in Framingham. J Chronic Dis 1967;20:511–24.
6. Jayes RL Jr, Beshansky JR, D'Agostino RB, et al. Do patients' coronary risk factor reports predict acute cardiac ischemia in the emergency department? A multicenter study. J Clin Epidemiol 1992;45(6):621–6.

7. Sievers J. Clinical features and outcome in three thousand thirty-six cases. Acta Med Scand 1964;406(Suppl):1–12.
8. Leven D. Chest pain-prophet of doom or nagging necrosis? Acta Med Scand 1981;644(Suppl):11–3.
9. Short D. Diagnosis of slight and subacute coronary attacks in the community. Br Heart J 1981;45:299–310.
10. Lee T, Cook E, Weisberg M, et al. Acute chest pain in the emergency room: identification and examination of low-risk patients. Arch Intern Med 1985;145:65–9.
11. Wilkinson K, Severance H. Identification of chest pain patients appropriate for an emergency department observation unit. Emerg Med Clin North Am 2001;19(1):35–66.
12. Swap CJ, Nagurney JT. Value and limitations of chest pain history in the evaluation of patients with suspected acute coronary syndrome. JAMA 2005;294(20):2623–9.
13. Fesmire FM, Wardton DR, Calhoun FB. Instability of ST segment sin the early stages of acute myocardial infarction in patients undergoing continuous 12-lead ECG monitoring. Am J Emerg Med 1995;13:158–63.
14. Fesmire FM, Bardoner JB. ST-segment instability preceding simultaneous cardiac arrest and AMI in a patient undergoing continuous 12-lead ECG monitoring. Am J Emerg Med 1994;12:69–76.
15. Fesmire FM, Percy RF, Wears RL, et al. Initial ECG in Qwave and non-Qwave myocardial infarction. Ann Emerg Med 1989;18:741–6.
16. Fesmire FM, Decker WW, Diercks DB, et al. Clinical policy: critical issue in the evaluation and management of adult patients with non-ST-segment elevation acute coronary syndromes. Ann Emerg Med 2006;48(3):272.
17. Kontos MC, Anderson FP, Schmidt KA, et al. Early diagnosis of acute myocardial infarction in patients without ST-segment elevation. Am J Cardiol 1999;83:155–8.
18. Apple FS, Anderson FP, Collinson P, et al. Clinical evaluation of the first medical whole blood, point-of-care testing device for detection of myocardial infarction. Clin Chem 2000;46:1604–9.
19. Gibler WB, Hoekstra JW, Weaver WD, et al. A randomized trial of the effects of early cardiac serum marker availability on reperfusion therapy in patients with acute myocardial infarction: the serial markers, acute myocardial infarction and rapid treatment trial (SMARTT). J Am Coll Cardiol 2000;36:1500–6.
20. Fesmire FM, Christenson RH, Fody EP, et al. Delta creatine kinase-MB outperforms myoglobin at two hours during the emergency department identification and exclusion of troponin positive non-ST-elevation acute coronary syndromes. Ann Emerg Med 2004;44:12–9.
21. Reichlin T, Hochholzer W, Bassetti S, et al. Early diagnosis of myocardial infarction with sensitive cardiac troponin assays. N Engl J Med 2009;361:858–67.
22. Yiadom MY, Kosowsky JM, Melanson SL, et al. Diagnostic performance of a highly sensitive cardiac troponin I assay in an emergency department setting. Clin Chem 2010;56(Suppl 6):A131.
23. Alcalai R, Planer D, Culhaoglu A, et al. Acute coronary syndrome vs nonspecific troponin elevation: clinical predictors and survival analysis. Arch Intern Med 2007;167:276–81.
24. Daly S, Campbell DA, Cameron PA. Short-stay units and observation medicine: a systematic review. Med J Aust 2003;178:559–63.
25. Martinez E, Reilly BM, Evans AT, et al. The observation unit: a new interface between inpatient and outpatient care. Am J Med 2001;110:274–7.

26. Anderson JL, Adams CD, Antman EM, et al. American College of Cardiology/American Heart Association 2007 guidelines for the management of patients with unstable angina/non-ST-elevation myocardial infarction: a report of the American College of Cardiology/American Heart Association Task Force on Practice Guidelines. J Am Coll Cardiol 2007;50:e1–157.

27. Chan GW, Sites FD, Shofer FS, et al. Impact of stress testing on 30-day cardiovascular outcomes for low-risk patients with chest pain admitted to floor telemetry beds. Am J Emerg Med 2003;21:282–7.

28. Mikhail MG, Smith FA, Gray M, et al. Cost-effectiveness of mandatory stress testing in chest pain center patients. Ann Emerg Med 1997;29:88–98.

29. Mair J, Smidt J, Lechleitner P, et al. A decision tree for the early diagnosis of acute myocardial infarction in nontraumatic chest pain patients at hospital admission. Chest 1995;108:1502–9.

30. Hilton TC, Thompson RC, Williams HJ, et al. Technetium-99m sestamibi myocardial perfusion imaging in the emergency room evaluation of chest pain. J Am Coll Cardiol 1994;23:1016–22.

31. Varetto T, Cantalupi D, Altieri A, et al. Emergency room technetium-99m sestamibi imaging to rule out acute myocardial ischemic events in patients with nondiagnostic electrocardiograms. J Am Coll Cardiol 1993;22:1804–8.

32. Amsterdam EA, Kirk JD, Diercks DB, et al. Exercise testing in chest pain units: rational, implementation, and results. Cardiol Clin 2005;23:503–16.

33. Fleischmann KE, Hunink MG, Kuntz KM, et al. Exercise echocardiography or exercise SPECT imaging? A meta-analysis of diagnostic test performance. JAMA 1998;280:913.

34. Gianrossi R, Detrano R, Mulvhill D, et al. Exercise-induced ST depression in the diagnosis of coronary artery disease: a meta-analysis. Circulation 1989;80:87.

35. Hoffman U, Ferencik M, Cury R, et al. Coronary CT angiography. J Nucl Med 2006;47:797–806.

Rhythm Disturbances

Allan R. Mottram, MD[a],*, James E. Svenson, MD[b]

KEYWORDS

- Dysrhythmia • Bradycardia • Supraventricular tachycardia
- Ventricular tachycardia

Patients with cardiac rhythm disturbances may present with a myriad of complaints ranging in severity from palpitations and weakness to chest pain and syncope. Patients may be unstable, requiring immediate interventions, or stable, allowing for a more deliberated approach. Rapid assessment of the patient's stability, underlying rhythm, and determination of appropriate interventions guides timely therapy.

Presenting rhythm disturbances may be primary dysrhythmias or may be secondary to an underlying medical problem. A critical step for the provider is to make this determination early, as this evaluation directly affects treatment. For example, a hypoxemic patient in respiratory failure with significant bradycardia requires attention to oxygenation and ventilation and will not benefit from pacing; a septic patient with sinus tachycardia will not benefit from cardioversion. Conversely, a patient with symptomatic bradycardia requires pharmacologic or electrical therapy to improve heart rate, and an unstable patient in atrial fibrillation with rapid ventricular response requires cardioversion. This article reviews the differential diagnosis and treatment of adult patients presenting with primary bradydysrhythmias and tachydysrhythmias, with the exception of atrial fibrillation and atrial flutter, which are covered in article by Bontempo and Goralnick elsewhere in this issue. A concise approach to diagnosis and determination of appropriate therapy is presented. Challenging scenarios are reviewed, for example, when the etiology of a dysrhythmia is unclear or complicated, as are safe and reliable interventions in such cases. Lastly, critical considerations for specific dysrhythmias are discussed, highlighting high-risk scenarios.

GENERAL APPROACH TO THE PATIENT WITH A CARDIAC RHYTHM DISTURBANCE

Identifying the rhythm disturbance as a primary problem rather than being secondary to a reversible underlying etiology is of critical importance. The use of the word

This work was not supported by any grant funding.
The authors have nothing to disclose.
[a] Division of Emergency Medicine, Department of Medicine, University of Wisconsin School of Medicine and Public Health, F2/204 CSC MC 3280, 600 Highland Avenue, Madison, WI 53792, USA
[b] Division of Emergency Medicine, Department of Medicine, University of Wisconsin School of Medicine and Public Health, F2/205 CSC MC 3280, 600 Highland Avenue, Madison, WI 53792, USA
* Corresponding author.
E-mail address: armottram@medicine.wisc.edu

Emerg Med Clin N Am 29 (2011) 729–746
doi:10.1016/j.emc.2011.08.007
0733-8627/11/$ – see front matter © 2011 Elsevier Inc. All rights reserved.

"primary" by the authors refers to those pathologies that are intrinsic to the heart, for example, acute myocardial infarction or infiltrative diseases resulting in bradycardia or accessory conduction pathways resulting in reentrant tachycardia. Primary rhythm disturbances may manifest as a result of abnormal impulse formation, ectopic electrical activity, or aberrant conduction. Dysrhythmias secondary to a reversible cause may manifest in the same way as primary rhythm disturbances. However, these patients will require interventions specific to the underlying etiology. The history and physical examination are invaluable for identifying the causes of primary or secondary arrhythmias, as outlined in **Table 1**. For example, patients with a known history of sinus node disease presenting with symptomatic bradycardia are likely to be in heart block, and those on rate-controlling medications are at risk for an adverse drug-related event resulting in bradycardia. Conversely, a patient with a history of supraventricular tachycardia (SVT) presenting with palpitations is likely to have had a recurrence. Physical examination findings consistent with a sepsis syndrome, frank pulmonary edema, or a patient with a history of missed dialysis might direct one away from a diagnosis of primary arrhythmia and toward a treatable underlying etiology. In the unstable patient the reversible causes outlined in **Table 2** must be considered before embarking on purely rhythm-based therapy.

A major determinant of stability in patients with bradycardic and tachycardic rhythm disturbances is heart rate. Patients with extremes of bradycardia and tachycardia will more likely present in an unstable condition, with such symptoms as altered mental status, syncope, dyspnea, chest pain, or cardiovascular collapse, and will require immediate intervention. Patients with impaired cardiovascular function at baseline will be less tolerant of such rhythms. Those with moderate bradycardias or tachycardias are more likely to have limited symptoms, to be hemodynamically normal, and allow time for deliberation and a focused approach to their care. This point is the first juncture in the approach to management of the patient with a primary dysrhythmia: is the patient stable or unstable (**Fig. 1**)? The stable patient allows time for a thorough evaluation and carefully tailored treatment; the unstable patient, defined as having altered mental status, hemodynamic instability, or chest pain considered to be of cardiac origin, requires emergent intervention.

Regardless of whether or not they are stable, all patients with symptomatic dysrhythmias require standard emergency evaluation and treatment. Such assessment includes evaluation of airway, breathing, and circulation with appropriate

Table 1 Potential causes of primary and secondary arrhythmias		
	Primary Arrhythmia	**Secondary Arrhythmia**
Bradycardic	Idiopathic Infiltrative disease Collagen vascular disease Ischemia or infarction Cardiac surgery Heritable arrhythmias Infectious disease (Lyme)	Autonomic syndromes Cardioactive drugs Hypothyroid Known comorbidities Reversible causes (see **Table 2**)
Tachycardic	Known prior dysrhythmia Structural heart disease Prior myocardial infarction	Autonomic syndromes Cardioactive drugs Hyperthyroid Known comorbidities Reversible causes (see **Table 2**)

Table 2 Reversible causes of arrhythmias	
Six H's	**Five T's**
Hypovolemia	Toxins
Hypoxia	Tamponade, cardiac
Hydrogen ion	Tension pneumothorax
Hypo-/hyperkalemia	Thrombosis
Hypoglycemia	Trauma
Hypothermia	

interventions as needed, supplementary oxygen, serial blood pressure monitoring, continuous cardiac rhythm monitoring, continuous pulse oximetry, intravenous access, and a 12-lead electrocardiogram (ECG), with additional testing and interventions as deemed necessary by the treating provider and as guided by the history and physical examination.

APPROACH TO THE PATIENT WITH A BRADYDYSRHYTHMIA
Evaluation

Bradycardia is defined as a heart rate less than 60 beats per minute (bpm). Many patients, such as highly trained athletes, tolerate bradycardia well and require no intervention. Pathologic bradycardias, on the other hand, result from either abnormal impulse formation or abnormal impulse conduction. The sinus node is dysfunctional in disorders of impulse formation, resulting in sinus bradycardia, sinus pause, or sinus arrest. With sinus pause of sufficient duration, and in sinus arrest, junctional or ventricular automaticity may result in slow escape rhythms with rates of roughly 40 to 60 or 30 to 40 bpm, respectively. In the absence of adequately conducted junctional or ventricular automaticity, asystole occurs. Abnormal impulse conduction may result in a variety of heart block conditions: intraventricular conduction delay, first-degree, second-degree type I, second-degree type II, and third-degree heart block. Intraventricular conduction delay and first-degree heart block are not expected to result in symptomatic bradycardia; however, they can confound rhythm interpretation, which is particularly true with bundle-branch blocks.

Interpretation of bradycardic dysrhythmias is relatively straightforward compared with interpretation of tachycardic dysrhythmias, due to the limited range of possibilities. **Box 1** provides a conceptual organization for basic bradycardic dysrhythmias. **Table 3** provides the ECG characteristics for sinus bradycardia and heart blocks

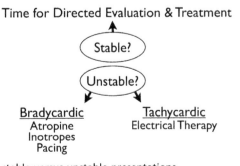

Fig. 1. Algorithm for stable versus unstable presentations.

Box 1
Conceptual approach to bradycardias

Regular, Narrow

Sinus bradycardia

Second degree type I

Slow atrial flutter

Junctional rhythms

Irregular, Narrow

Slow atrial fibrillation

Slow atrial flutter

Slow multifocal atrial tachycardia

Second degree type I or II

Third degree

Regular, Wide

Sinus bradycardia aberrancy

Irregular, Wide

Idioventricular rhythm

Atrial fibrillation/flutter with aberrancy

Heart block with aberrancy

---

without aberrant conduction as well as important causes to consider during acute presentation of these primary dysrhythmias. Note that the differential diagnosis is not limited to these important causes. Acute coronary syndrome must be considered in all patients presenting with a bradyarrhythmia. Brady and colleagues[1] described

---

Table 3
Characteristics of bradycardia and heart block

	Sinus Bradycardia	First-Degree Block	Second-Degree Type I Block	Second-Degree Type II Block	Third-Degree Block
Atrial rate	≤60	Any	Any	Any	Any
Ventricular rate	Matches atrial rate	Matches atrial rate	Slower than atrial rate	Slower than atrial rate	Slower than atrial rate
Rhythm	Regular, P-QRS ratio 1:1	Regular, P-QRS ratio 1:1	Irregular	Regular or Irregular	Irregular
PR	<200 ms	≥200 ms	**Prolongs before dropped QRS**	**Fixed before dropped QRS**	**No association**
Acute causes to consider	Normal drugs Vagal tone ACS	Drugs Vasovagal ACS	Drugs Vagal tone ACS	ACS	ACS

Key characteristics are in boldface.
Abbreviation: ACS, acute coronary syndrome.

a case series of 131 patients presenting with unstable bradycardia and heart block, all of whom received atropine and some of whom were paced. Of these, 45 (34%) had a discharge diagnosis of myocardial infarction and 12 (9%) had a discharge diagnosis of ischemia. Of the 45 presenting with atrioventricular (AV) block, 25 (56%) had a discharge diagnosis of myocardial infarction.

Treatment

Stable bradydysrhythmias

The stable patient with asymptomatic bradycardia may be observed, without any specific emergent intervention. For example, a patient with bradycardia due to third-degree heart block may present in stable condition and without symptoms while at rest, though he or she may complain of exertional dyspnea, weakness, or dizziness while ambulating. Such a patient requires hospitalization for evaluation and management of the heart block; however, emergency interventions such as atropine, inotrope infusion, or pacing are not indicated.

Unstable bradydysrhythmias

Atropine is the first-line treatment for symptomatic bradycardia, a recommendation that is supported by consensus opinion as well as research performed in the prehospital setting, emergency department, and operating room.[1–5] The initial dose is 0.5 mg as an intravenous bolus, and may be repeated every 3 to 5 minutes to a maximum of 3 mg. Atropine may prove adequate as a sole intervention, with the patient only requiring further monitoring.

However, if it is ineffective or if recurrent doses of atropine are required, transcutaneous pacing or inotrope infusion should be considered. As with the recommendation for atropine as a first-line agent, consensus and limited scientific evidence support the use of pacing or inotrope infusion as equally effective second-line interventions after atropine.[2–5] The recommended inotropes are dopamine, 2 to 10 μg/kg/min or epinephrine, 2 to 10 μg/min.[3] **Fig. 2** provides a framework for treating the patient with symptomatic bradycardia. Transcutaneous pacing requires sedation and analgesia in the conscious patient, whereas inotrope infusion does not. In all patients, but especially those who do not respond promptly and adequately to atropine, preparations for transvenous pacing should be initiated. Once the patient is stabilized the provider should again review the potential etiology, with particular attention to identifying reversible causes of the abnormal presenting rhythm.

APPROACH TO THE PATIENT WITH A TACHYDYSRHYTHMIA

Evaluation

Tachycardia is defined as a heart rate greater than 100 bpm. Tachycardia is more likely to be a primary arrhythmia when the heart rate exceeds 150 bpm. The upper rate of sinus tachycardia can be approximated by subtracting the patient's age in years from 220. Because a rapid heart rate is often an appropriate response to a physiologic stress such as fever, dehydration, or anemia, such factors should be identified early to determine whether the rate is a primary dysrhythmia or secondary to an underlying condition, with treatment aimed at the underlying cause if present. For example, when cardiac output and systemic perfusion are dependent on heart rate, as in the septic patient, slowing the heart rate may be detrimental. However, when the etiology of sinus tachycardia is not correctable with intravenous volume, analgesics, or anxiolytics, limiting the tachycardic response and, therefore, myocardial oxygen consumption, may be desirable in select critically ill patients.[6]

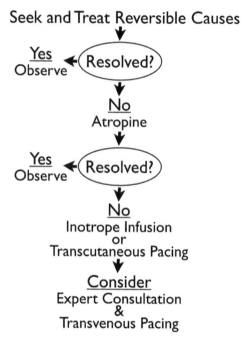

Fig. 2. Approach to treatment of symptomatic bradycardias.

Tachydysrhythmias may be classified based on the regularity of the rhythm and the width of the QRS complex (**Box 2**). Those with a QRS duration less than 120 milliseconds are considered narrow complex tachycardias, with the origin above the bundle of His. When the duration of the QRS complex is greater than 120 milliseconds, the rhythm is considered a wide complex tachycardia. Irregular narrow complex tachydysrhythmias include atrial fibrillation, atrial tachycardia, atrial flutter with variable AV conduction, and multifocal atrial tachycardia. Regular tachydysrhythmias include sinus tachycardia, atrial flutter, atrial tachycardia, AV nodal reentry tachycardia, and AV reentrant tachycardia. Note that some tachydysrhythmias may be regular or irregular, such as atrial flutter. Regular wide complex tachydysrhythmias are generally considered to be ventricular tachycardia or SVT with aberrancy; however, antidromic AV reentrant tachycardia (AVRT) may present as a wide complex tachycardia. Irregular wide complex tachycardias may be polymorphic ventricular tachycardia or an irregular supraventricular rhythm with an abnormal conduction path. Examples of this latter phenomenon include atrial fibrillation, atrial flutter with variable conduction, or atrial tachycardia with variable conduction, in the setting of bundle-branch block or conduction via an accessory pathway such as with Wolfe-Parkinson-White syndrome. Care should be taken to evaluate such rhythms on a 12-lead ECG when possible, as a wide complex tachycardia may appear narrow on a single-lead rhythm strip.[7]

Narrow complex tachydysrhythmias

Narrow complex tachydysrhythmias include sinus tachycardia, atrial flutter, atrial fibrillation, AV nodal reentrant tachycardia (AVNRT), orthodromic AVRT, atrial tachycardia, multifocal atrial tachycardia, and junctional tachycardia. Though atrial fibrillation and flutter are types of SVT, they are reviewed elsewhere in this issue and are not discussed further here.

Box 2
Conceptual approach to tachycardias

Regular, Narrow

1. Sinus tachycardia

2. Atrial flutter

3. Atrial tachycardia

4. AV nodal reentrant tachycardia

5. AV reentrant tachycardia

6. Junctional tachycardia

Irregular, Narrow

1. Atrial fibrillation

2. Atrial tachycardia—variable conduction

3. Atrial flutter—variable conduction

4. Multifocal atrial tachycardia

Regular, Wide

1. Supraventricular tachycardia with aberrancy

2. Ventricular tachycardia

Irregular, Wide

1. Above rhythms with either

a. Aberrancy

b. Accessory pathway

2. Polymorphic ventricular tachycardia

AVNRT is the most common type of nonatrial fibrillation/flutter SVT in adults, with AVRT being the second most common.[8] The cause of AVNRT is a reentrant pathway or tract within the AV node, which appears as a regular, narrow SVT on the electrocardiogram. AVRT is caused by the presence of an abnormal accessory pathway that serves as a conduit for impulses that originate from the sinoatrial node and allows more rapid conduction, bypassing the AV node either on its way to the ventricles (antidromic) or on its return to the atria (orthodromic). The result is a reentrant circuit such as that seen in Wolff-Parkinson-White syndrome.[9] **Fig. 3** provides a visual summary of this concept. In patients with orthodromic AVRT, the tachydysrhythmia may appear as a regular narrow complex SVT indistinguishable from AVNRT. Antidromic AVRT appears as a regular wide complex tachycardia on ECG and may be indistinguishable from ventricular tachycardia, especially if the clinical history of a bypass tract is not known.

Atrial tachycardia is an SVT that can originate from a single focus of atrial tissue or be multifocal in origin, and is the result of increased automaticity.[10,11] Atrial tachycardia can be either focal or macro-reentrant. In focal atrial tachycardia, atrial activation starts rhythmically in a small area from which it spreads out centrifugally. In macro-reentry, reentrant activation occurs around a central obstacle; this would include, for example, typical atrial flutter.[11] Multifocal atrial tachycardia is defined as a rhythm with an atrial rate greater than 100 bpm, at least 3 morphologically distinct P waves, irregular P-P intervals, and an isoelectric baseline between P waves.[12]

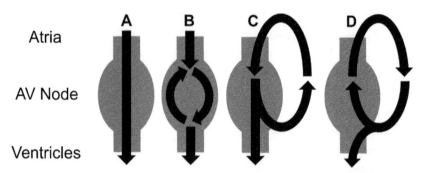

Atria

AV Node

Ventricles

Fig. 3. Conduction through the atrioventricular (AV) node in sinus rhythm and paroxysmal supraventricular tachycardia. (*A*) Sinus rhythm; (*B*) atrioventricular nodal reentry tachycardia; (*C*) orthodromic atrioventricular reentry tachycardia; (*D*) antidromic atrioventricular reentry tachycardia.

Junctional tachycardia is also a disorder of increased automaticity, although it is relatively rare. It is approached in a manner similar to the atrial tachycardias.

Wide complex tachydysrhythmias

Differentiating between ventricular tachycardia and SVT with aberrant conduction can be challenging, and the rhythm should be assumed to be ventricular tachycardia in the absence of clear-cut evidence to the contrary. Clinical findings that support the diagnosis of ventricular tachycardia include symptoms consistent with myocardial infarction or ischemia, prior myocardial infarction or coronary artery disease, and symptoms occurring in older patients.[13] Hemodynamic stability should not be used to discriminate between ventricular tachycardia and SVT with aberrancy.[14] Factors associated with the diagnosis of SVT with aberrancy include young patients, prior bundle-branch block or similar appearance on prior electrocardiogram, and a history of SVT with aberrancy. Several decision rules have been proposed in attempts to identify features on the ECG to differentiate ventricular tachycardia from SVT with aberrancy. Brugada and colleagues[15] proposed a simplified algorithm based on 4 criteria applied in a stepwise manner: absence of RS in all precordial leads; R to S interval greater than 100 milliseconds in one precordial lead; AV dissociation; and morphologic criteria for ventricular tachycardia present in V1, V2, and V6. The criteria are designed to be applied in a stepwise manner, and if at any step criteria are present the diagnosis is ventricular tachycardia. If none are present the rhythm is determined to be SVT with aberrancy. These investigators prospectively applied their criteria and demonstrated a sensitivity and specificity of 98.7% and 96.5%, respectively, for correctly identifying ventricular tachycardia. Other investigators have found the Brugada criteria to be useful, though not as reliable as reported by Brugada and colleagues, and have proposed alterative approaches.[16–18] Overall, although algorithmic approaches to identifying the etiology of wide complex tachycardias are helpful, there are a substantial number of cases where even expert electrocardiogram analysis is indeterminate.[17]

Treatment

Unstable narrow complex tachydysrhythmias

Management of the adult patient presenting with an unstable tachydysrhythmia can be relatively straightforward if certain fundamental decision points are considered and acted on appropriately, as outlined in **Fig. 4**. The critical actions are the following: assess patient stability, identify and treat underlying causes if present, identify the

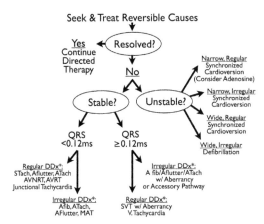

Fig. 4. Approach the patient with tachycardia. Note the emergent interventions for unstable rhythms and the differential diagnosis for stable rhythms. * Readers are referred to the text for discussion of interventions for stable tachydysrhythmias. Afib, atrial fibrillation; Aflutter, atrial flutter; ATach, atrial tachycardia; AVNRT, atrioventricular nodal reentry tachycardia; AVRT, atrioventricular reentry tachycardia; DDx, differential diagnosis; MAT, multifocal atrial tachycardia; STach, sinus tachycardia; SVT, supraventricular tachycardia; w/, with.

heart rate, rhythm, and QRS morphology, and select electrical and/or pharmacologic interventions. Unstable patients, for example, those with a systolic blood pressure less than 90 mm Hg, chest pain, or altered mental status, with a narrow complex SVT that is not a compensatory sinus tachycardia, should be immediately cardioverted. Cardioversion of nonatrial fibrillation SVT can be successful with low energies, from 50 to 100 J when using a biphasic defibrillator, and 200 J when using monophasic defibrillator.[3,19] If the initial cardioversion fails, then the dose should be increased in a stepwise fashion.[20] Although the current American Heart Association guidelines generally recommend synchronized cardioversion as the treatment of choice for all unstable tachydysrhythmias, a trial of adenosine may be considered in patients with mildly unstable narrow complex regular SVT before cardioversion.[3] This recommendation is based on retrospective evidence showing that adenosine may convert unstable narrow complex SVT promptly and resolve hemodynamic instability.[21–25]

Stable narrow complex tachydysrhythmias

The differential diagnosis for stable narrow complex supraventricular rhythms is discussed above. For the purposes of this article, discussion of specific interventions is limited to those for AVNRT, AVRT, and atrial tachycardias, excluding atrial fibrillation and atrial flutter. The goal in treatment of these tachydysrhythmias is rate and rhythm control. For AVNRT and AVRT, as opposed to disorders of atrial automaticity, the distinguishing feature is a reentry circuit involving the AV node. Both AVNRT and orthodromic AVRT (jointly referred to as SVT for the remainder of the article) will present as narrow complex regular tachycardias. Regular, stable, monomorphic, wide complex tachycardias in the setting of known preexisting bundle-branch block that do not meet criteria for ventricular tachycardia may also be supraventricular in origin. Similarly, antidromic AVRT will present as a regular wide complex tachydysrhythmia. Discussion of these more complicated wide complex tachyarrhythmias is expanded in the section on stable wide complex tachycardia.

The approach to treating SVT is relatively straightforward and may involve either vagal maneuvers, adenosine, or nodal blocking agents (calcium-channel blockers or β-blockers). Vagal maneuvers and adenosine are the preferred initial interventions. The most widely used vagal maneuver is the Valsalva maneuver, with a success rate of approximately 15% to 20%.[26] However, success rates of up to 30% have been reported using a modified Valsalva maneuver whereby patients expired into a section of suction tubing and pressure gauge for at least 15 seconds at 40 mm Hg while in a Trendelenburg position.[27] Carotid massage may be considered. As a diagnostic tool it may slow the ventricular rate to assist in rhythm analysis, and as a therapeutic tool it is equivalent to Valsalva in terminating SVT.[28] However, concerns have been raised regarding the safety of carotid massage especially in the elderly, with neurologic complications being reported in 0.1% to 1%.[29,30]

Adenosine is the second-line agent if SVT does not respond to vagal maneuvers, and has several advantages over other agents. For example, it demonstrates similar conversion rates to calcium-channel blockers with the advantage of a more rapid onset and fewer side effects. It has a short half-life, which allows for use of other AV nodal blocking agents if necessary.[31–33] Adenosine is administered as a rapid intravenous bolus, with an initial dose of 6 mg. If the rhythm does not convert, the dose should be increased to 12 mg and repeated. Common side effects are flushing, dyspnea, and chest discomfort.[34] Bronchospasm has been reported following adenosine administration in patients with underlying asthma or chronic obstructive pulmonary disease; however, it has also been reported to be given safely in such cases, and as such is a relative contraindication.[26,35] Patients treated with adenosine may convert to a different arrhythmia, including prolonged AV block, paroxysmal atrial fibrillation, nonventricular tachycardia, transient premature ventricular complexes, torsades de pointes, atrial fibrillation, or atrial flutter, with such conversions being noted to occur in 13% of patients.[34] Most of these arrhythmias are transient and recover spontaneously. When an underlying preexcitation syndrome such as Wolff-Parkinson-White is suspected despite a presentation with a narrow complex regular tachycardia, a defibrillator should be available out of concern for the possibility of inducing atrial fibrillation with rapid ventricular response.

When SVT fails to convert to sinus rhythm, recurs, or when treatment with vagal maneuvers or adenosine reveal atrial fibrillation or atrial flutter, treatment with AV nodal blocking agents is indicated. These agents include the nondihydropyridine calcium-channel blockers verapamil and diltiazem, and β-blockers. Verapamil and diltiazem have similar efficacy in the treatment of narrow complex SVT, though they have a more concerning side effect profile when compared with adenosine.[31,33,36–39] Verapamil and diltiazem should only be used in cases known to be supraventricular in origin, and they should avoided in patients with reduced left ventricular function. All nodal blocking agents should be avoided in patients with wide complex tachycardias, preexcited atrial fibrillation, or atrial flutter. The initial dose of verapamil is 5 mg, administered intravenously. If there is no response and no drug-related side effects, the dose can be repeated every 15 minutes up to a total of 20 to 30 mg. The initial dose for diltiazem is 20 mg, and an additional 20 mg may be administered as needed after 15 minutes. A diltiazem maintenance infusion at 5 to 15 mg/h may be used if continuous rate control is required.[3] Pretreatment with 1 g calcium gluconate or 333 mg calcium chloride has been suggested as an intervention to act against hypotension during calcium-channel blocker use.[40]

β-Blockers slow conduction through the AV node and reduce sympathetic tone. Though suggested as second-line agent for SVT, the evidence supporting their use is more limited.[41–45] Like calcium-channel blockers they have a significant side-effect profile in this setting, including bradycardia, conduction delays, and hypotension. Furthermore, they are less effective when compared with calcium-channel blockers.[46,47] Serial use of these long acting AV nodal blocking drugs should be avoided, as hypotension and bradycardia are a significant risk.[3] Alternative drug therapy includes antiarrhythmic agents such as amiodarone, procainamide, or sotalol. However, these drugs have potential for toxicity and proarrhythmic effects, and as such their use in SVT is limited.

Lastly, atrial tachycardia and multifocal atrial tachycardia are considered. These disorders are of increased automaticity at a single or multiple atrial sites, respectively. These conditions differ from SVT in that the ectopic electrical activity resides in the atria, and there is no reentrant circuit through the AV node. Multifocal atrial tachycardia is typically an epiphenomenon of an underlying disorder such as hypoxemia, chronic obstructive pulmonary disease, congestive heart failure, and electrolyte disorders.[10] Reversal of precipitating causes remains the cornerstone of treatment for multifocal atrial tachycardia, as this may be all that is required to control the arrhythmia and avoid the potentially harmful effects of antiarrhythmic agents. If the arrhythmia persists, the clinical significance of the tachycardia must be evaluated before the use of antiarrhythmics is considered. Because they are disorders of automaticity, electrical cardioversion is not effective and pharmacologic therapy is required. Agents to consider are β-blockers, calcium-channel blockers, and amiodarone. Metoprolol has been shown to be effective for rate control in a double-blind, placebo-controlled trial, and may be considered a first line in the treatment of multifocal atrial tachycardia in the absence of contraindications.[48,49] However, in patients with impaired left ventricular function, drugs with negative inotropic properties should be avoided. In such cases amiodarone may be preferred.[50,51]

Unstable wide complex tachydysrhythmias

Synchronized cardioversion is recommended for unstable monomorphic ventricular tachycardia when a pulse is present, with initial energies of 100 J whether using a biphasic or monophasic defibrillator. Pulseless ventricular tachycardia is treated the same as ventricular fibrillation, and is defibrillated. The initial energy is 120 to 200 J for biphasic defibrillators based on the manufacturer's recommendation, or 360 J for monophasic defibrillators. Unstable wide irregular tachycardias should also be treated with defibrillation using the same energy setting.

Polymorphic ventricular tachycardia presents as an irregular wide complex tachycardia with varying QRS morphology. It is typically associated with hemodynamic instability, and often degenerates to ventricular fibrillation. As outlined earlier, the treatment of choice for such unstable patients is defibrillation with the same strategy as for ventricular fibrillation, and attention to identifying and treating the underlying cause of the dysrhythmia.[3] Efforts should be directed to identifying and treating ischemia, electrolyte abnormalities, or drug toxicities that may have precipitated the arrhythmia. For patients who have experienced polymorphic ventricular tachycardia without a prolonged QT interval, the most common cause is myocardial ischemia. In such cases, when the dysrhythmia has resolved, β-blockers are appropriate, amiodarone may be effective in preventing arrhythmia recurrence, and prompt percutaneous coronary intervention should be considered.[3] Less common causes of polymorphic ventricular tachycardia include Brugada syndrome and catecholaminergic ventricular tachycardia, which may be responsive to isoproterenol and β-blockers, respectively. However, expert consultation is advised.

Polymorphic ventricular tachycardia may or may not be torsades de pointes, and this cannot be distinguished on the ECG during a period of ventricular tachycardia.

Torsades de pointes is diagnosed when a prolonged QT interval is known to be present or is observed during a period of sinus rhythm. It is often preceded by a period of bradycardia, and is more likely to occur in the setting of electrolyte abnormalities or when preceded by a QT-prolonging antiarrhythmic infusion such as procainamide, quinidine, or sotolol. Whether torsades de pointes is due to a congenital long-QT syndrome or if it is acquired, the management approach is similar. Magnesium infusion of 1 to 2 g over 15 minutes may be effective.[52–54] In patients with recurrent polymorphic ventricular tachycardia accompanied by bradycardia or precipitated by pauses in rhythm, temporary overdrive pacing is appropriate.[55] Similarly, isoproterenol may be an effective treatment in drug-induced QT prolongation by increasing heart rate and shortening the QT interval.[56] However, it should be avoided in patients with suspected ischemia because it increases myocardial oxygen demand, as well as in patients with congenital long-QT syndromes. QT-prolonging drugs should be recognized and discontinued, and electrolyte abnormalities should be corrected.

Stable wide complex tachydysrhythmias

As in stable narrow complex tachycardia, the first step in management is to determine whether the rhythm is regular or irregular. A regular wide complex tachycardia is either ventricular tachycardia, SVT with aberrant conduction (AVNRT with aberrancy or orthodromic AVRT with aberrancy), or antidromic AVRT. Irregular wide complex tachycardias may be atrial fibrillation with aberrancy, preexcited atrial fibrillation, or polymorphic ventricular tachycardia (torsades de pointes). A very rapid (>220 bpm) irregular wide complex tachycardia is virtually pathognomonic of preexcited atrial fibrillation.[57]

If the origin of a stable, regular, monomorphic wide complex tachycardia cannot be determined, adenosine has been demonstrated to be safe and effective for diagnostic and therapeutic purposes.[58] Furthermore, the likelihood of making a correct diagnosis of SVT or ventricular tachycardia increases. If the underlying rhythm is SVT with aberrant conduction, administration of adenosine will likely result in conversion to sinus rhythm.[58] If the rhythm is ventricular tachycardia there will likely be no effect, although there is a subset of patients with ventricular tachycardia responsive to adenosine.[59] Adenosine should not be used in irregular or polymorphic ventricular tachycardia. The treating provider should be prepared for defibrillation under such circumstances.

Given the diagnostic uncertainty often seen in cases of wide complex tachycardia, the default should be to treat such rhythms as ventricular tachycardia unless there is clear evidence to the contrary.[60] Cardioversion or antiarrhythmic drugs are the recommended treatment strategy. Cardioversion is a safe, rapidly effective intervention with relatively few side effects even in the setting of stable ventricular dysrhythmias. When a pharmacologic approach is desired, the recommended drugs include procainamide, amiodarone, and sotolol. Procainamide and sotolol should be avoided in cases of prolonged QT interval. In cases where one pharmacologic agent has not been effective, cardioversion should be attempted or expert consultation obtained before administration of a second pharmacologic agent.[3]

Procainamide is the preferred pharmacologic agent for treatment of hemodynamically stable ventricular tachycardia when cardioversion is not selected as the first-line intervention. Procainamide has a relatively fast onset of action and terminates ventricular tachycardia in to 80% to 90% of patients.[61] Procainamide is recommended as an infusion of 20 to 50 mg/min to a total dose of 17 mg/kg. The other end points are arrhythmia suppression, hypotension, or QRS duration increase of greater than 50%. Hypotension is more common with higher infusion rates.[62] Procainamide should be avoided in patients with reduced left ventricular function, congestive heart failure, or prolonged QT interval. Although procainamide may be more effective than amiodarone in the short term, it should be noted that no difference has been demonstrated in treating sustained ventricular tachycardia, and that amiodarone is the preferred agent in patients with reduced left ventricular function.[50,63]

Amiodarone has proved useful in hemodynamically unstable and recurrent ventricular tachycardia.[64,65] Some studies have demonstrated it to be effective in hemodynamically unstable patients with monomorphic ventricular tachycardia refractory to other medications, whereas others have shown that it is no more effective than other antiarrhythmics.[66–68] Care should be taken to monitor for hypotension, although it is thought that this adverse effect was attributable to the solvent used in older formulations of the drug.[69] The dose of amiodarone is 150 mg over 10 minutes repeated to a maximum of 2.2 g over 24 hours.

Sotalol is much less commonly used in emergency medicine practice, although it has been used with success to treat stable sustained monomorphic ventricular tachycardia, and has been demonstrated to be more effective than lidocaine.[70,71] The dose of sotalol is 100 mg (1.5 mg/kg) given over 5 minutes.

Although management of atrial fibrillation is discussed elsewhere, the special case of atrial fibrillation with AVRT (Wolff-Parkinson-White syndrome) is mentioned here, as it is in the differential for wide complex tachycardias and has specific management considerations. AV nodal blocking agents used for most supraventricular rhythms (adenosine, calcium-channel blockers, β-blockers) should be avoided in this circumstance. These agents slow conduction through the AV node, but do not affect conduction through the accessory pathway, which can allow very rapid conduction of up to 300 to 400 bpm.[72] In such cases AV nodal blocking agents may accelerate conduction over the accessory pathway, resulting in cardiovascular decompensation and ventricular fibrillation.[73,74] In general, patients with preexcited atrial fibrillation are unstable, with very rapid heart rates, and require emergent cardioversion. Pharmacologic interventions should be approached with great caution, and only in cases where cardioversion is not appropriate or effective.[3] Agents to consider include procainamide and amiodarone. Procainamide increases the antegrade effective refractory period and the intra-atrial conduction time.[75] Schatz and colleagues[76] support procainamide as the favored pharmacologic treatment for patients with preexcited atrial fibrillation, due to its ability to safely lengthen the effective refractory period. Amiodarone may be effective, but recent studies have shown a small yet serious risk of ventricular fibrillation in this setting.[77–81] The use of either amiodarone or procainamide may also result in the termination of the atrial rhythm, as such thromboembolic complications must be considered.

SUMMARY

Patients with cardiac rhythm disturbances can be challenging to manage, especially when they present under emergent conditions. High-quality, safe emergency care involves rapid assessment focusing on identification of the unstable patient, recognition of comorbidities, dysrhythmia diagnosis, and prompt intervention. A useful cognitive strategy is to categorize patients as stable or unstable, and the rhythm as fast or slow, regular or irregular, and wide or narrow. The differential diagnosis is hence narrowed, and focused interventions can be selected in a rapid, informed, and organized manner.

REFERENCES

1. Brady WJ, Swart G, DeBehnke DJ, et al. The efficacy of atropine in the treatment of hemodynamically unstable bradycardia and atrioventricular block: prehospital and emergency department considerations. Resuscitation 1999;41:47–55.

2. Morrison LJ, Deakin CD, Morley PT, et al. Part 8: advanced life support: 2010 International Consensus on Cardiopulmonary Resuscitation and Emergency Cardiovascular Care Science With Treatment Recommendations. Circulation 2010;122:S345–421.

3. Neumar RW, Otto CW, Link MS, et al. Part 8: adult advanced cardiovascular life support: 2010 American Heart Association Guidelines for Cardiopulmonary Resuscitation and Emergency Cardiovascular Care. Circulation 2010;122: S729–67.

4. Morrison LJ, Long J, Vermeulen M, et al. A randomized controlled feasibility trial comparing safety and effectiveness of prehospital pacing versus conventional treatment: 'PrePACE'. Resuscitation 2008;76:341–9.

5. Smith I, Monk TG, White PF. Comparison of transesophageal atrial pacing with anticholinergic drugs for the treatment of intraoperative bradycardia. Anesth Analg 1994;78:245–52.

6. Gabrielli A, Gallagher TJ, Caruso LJ, et al. Diltiazem to treat sinus tachycardia in critically ill patients: a four-year experience. Crit Care Med 2001;29:1874–9.

7. Hood RE, Shorofsky SR. Management of arrhythmias in the emergency department. Cardiol Clin 2006;24:125–33, vii.

8. Porter MJ, Morton JB, Denman R, et al. Influence of age and gender on the mechanism of supraventricular tachycardia. Heart Rhythm 2004;1:393–6.

9. Mark DG, Brady WJ, Pines JM. Preexcitation syndromes: diagnostic consideration in the ED. Am J Emerg Med 2009;27:878–88.

10. McCord J, Borzak S. Multifocal atrial tachycardia. Chest 1998;113:203–9.

11. Roberts-Thomson KC, Kistler PM, Kalman JM. Atrial tachycardia: mechanisms, diagnosis, and management. Curr Probl Cardiol 2005;30:529–73.

12. Shine KI, Kastor JA, Yurchak PM. Multifocal atrial tachycardia. Clinical and electrocardiographic features in 32 patients. N Engl J Med 1968;279:344–9.

13. Wellens HJ. Electrophysiology: ventricular tachycardia: diagnosis of broad QRS complex tachycardia. Heart 2001;86:579–85.

14. Steinman RT, Herrera C, Schuger CD, et al. Wide QRS tachycardia in the conscious adult. Ventricular tachycardia is the most frequent cause. JAMA 1989;261:1013–6.

15. Brugada P, Brugada J, Mont L, et al. A new approach to the differential diagnosis of a regular tachycardia with a wide QRS complex. Circulation 1991;83:1649–59.

16. Alberca T, Almendral J, Sanz P, et al. Evaluation of the specificity of morphological electrocardiographic criteria for the differential diagnosis of wide QRS complex tachycardia in patients with intraventricular conduction defects. Circulation 1997;96:3527–33.

17. Drew BJ, Scheinman MM. ECG criteria to distinguish between aberrantly conducted supraventricular tachycardia and ventricular tachycardia: practical aspects for the immediate care setting. Pacing Clin Electrophysiol 1995;18: 2194–208.

18. Vereckei A, Duray G, Szénási G, et al. Application of a new algorithm in the differential diagnosis of wide QRS complex tachycardia. Eur Heart J 2007;28:589–600.

19. Link MS, Atkins DL, Passman RS, et al. Part 6: electrical therapies: automated external defibrillators, defibrillation, cardioversion, and pacing: 2010 American Heart Association Guidelines for Cardiopulmonary Resuscitation and Emergency Cardiovascular Care. Circulation 2010;122:S706–19.

20. Singh SN, Tang XC, Reda D, et al. Systematic electrocardioversion for atrial fibrillation and role of antiarrhythmic drugs: a substudy of the SAFE-T trial. Heart Rhythm 2009;6:152–5.

21. Gausche M, Persse DE, Sugarman T, et al. Adenosine for the prehospital treatment of paroxysmal supraventricular tachycardia. Ann Emerg Med 1994;24: 183–9.
22. Losek JD, Endom E, Dietrich A, et al. Adenosine and pediatric supraventricular tachycardia in the emergency department: multicenter study and review. Ann Emerg Med 1999;33:185–91.
23. Marco CA, Cardinale JF. Adenosine for the treatment of supraventricular tachycardia in the ED. Am J Emerg Med 1994;12:485–8.
24. McCabe JL, Adhar GC, Menegazzi JJ, et al. Intravenous adenosine in the prehospital treatment of paroxysmal supraventricular tachycardia. Ann Emerg Med 1992;21:358–61.
25. Melio FR, Mallon WK, Newton EH. Successful conversion of unstable supraventricular tachycardia to sinus rhythm with adenosine. Ann Emerg Med 1993;22: 709–13.
26. Lim SH, Anantharaman V, Teo WS, et al. Comparison of treatment of supraventricular tachycardia by Valsalva maneuver and carotid sinus massage. Ann Emerg Med 1998;31:30–5.
27. Walker S, Cutting P. Impact of a modified Valsalva manoeuvre in the termination of paroxysmal supraventricular tachycardia. Emerg Med J 2010;27:287–91.
28. Adlington H, Cumberbatch G. Carotid sinus massage: is it a safe way to terminate supraventricular tachycardia? Emerg Med J 2009;26:459.
29. Walsh KA, Ezri MD, Denes P. Emergency treatment of tachyarrhythmias. Med Clin North Am 1986;70:791–811.
30. Walsh T, Clinch D, Costelloe A, et al. Carotid sinus massage—how safe is it? Age Ageing 2006;35:518–20.
31. Brady WJ, DeBehnke DJ, Wickman LL, et al. Treatment of out-of-hospital supraventricular tachycardia: adenosine vs verapamil. Acad Emerg Med 1996;3: 574–85.
32. DiMarco JP, Miles W, Akhtar M, et al. Adenosine for paroxysmal supraventricular tachycardia: dose ranging and comparison with verapamil. Assessment in placebo-controlled, multicenter trials. The Adenosine for PSVT Study Group. Ann Intern Med 1990;113:104–10.
33. Holdgate A, Foo A. Adenosine versus intravenous calcium channel antagonists for the treatment of supraventricular tachycardia in adults. Cochrane Database Syst Rev 2006;4:CD005154.
34. Innes JA. Review article: adenosine use in the emergency department. Emerg Med Australas 2008;20:209–15.
35. Terry P, Lumsden G. Towards evidence based emergency medicine: best BETs from the Manchester Royal Infirmary. Using intravenous adenosine in asthmatics. Emerg Med J 2001;18:61.
36. Boudonas G, Lefkos N, Efthymiadis AP, et al. Intravenous administration of diltiazem in the treatment of supraventricular tachyarrhythmias. Acta Cardiol 1995;50: 125–34.
37. Cheiman DM, Shea BF, Kelly RA. Treatment of supraventricular tachyarrhythmias with intravenous calcium channel blockers: are subtle differences worth the cost? Pharmacotherapy 1996;16:861–8.
38. Lim SH, Anantharaman V, Teo WS. Slow-infusion of calcium channel blockers in the emergency management of supraventricular tachycardia. Resuscitation 2002;52:167–74.
39. Seth S, Mittal A, Goel P, et al. Low-dose intravenous diltiazem—efficacy and safety in supraventricular tachyarrhythmias. Indian Heart J 1996;48:365–7.

40. Jameson SJ, Hargarten SW. Calcium pretreatment to prevent verapamil-induced hypotension in patients with SVT. Ann Emerg Med 1992;21:68.
41. Amsterdam EA, Kulcyski J, Ridgeway MG. Efficacy of cardioselective beta-adrenergic blockade with intravenously administered metoprolol in the treatment of supraventricular tachyarrhythmias. J Clin Pharmacol 1991;31:714–8.
42. Das G, Ferris J. Esmolol in the treatment of supraventricular tachyarrhythmias. Can J Cardiol 1988;4:177–80.
43. Das G, Tschida V, Gray R, et al. Efficacy of esmolol in the treatment and transfer of patients with supraventricular tachyarrhythmias to alternate oral antiarrhythmic agents. J Clin Pharmacol 1988;28:746–50.
44. Morganroth J, Horowitz LN, Anderson J, et al. Comparative efficacy and tolerance of esmolol to propranolol for control of supraventricular tachyarrhythmia. Am J Cardiol 1985;56:33F–9F.
45. Rehnqvist N. Clinical experience with intravenous metoprolol in supraventricular tachyarrhythmias. A multicentre study. Ann Clin Res 1981;13(Suppl 30): 68–72.
46. Gupta A, Naik A, Vora A, et al. Comparison of efficacy of intravenous diltiazem and esmolol in terminating supraventricular tachycardia. J Assoc Physicians India 1999;47:969–72.
47. Komatsu C, Ishinaga T, Tateishi O, et al. Effects of four antiarrhythmic drugs on the induction and termination of paroxysmal supraventricular tachycardia. Jpn Circ J 1986;50:961–72.
48. Arsura E, Lefkin AS, Scher DL, et al. A randomized, double-blind, placebo-controlled study of verapamil and metoprolol in treatment of multifocal atrial tachycardia. Am J Med 1988;85:519–24.
49. Arsura EL, Solar M, Lefkin AS, et al. Metoprolol in the treatment of multifocal atrial tachycardia. Crit Care Med 1987;15:591–4.
50. Kudenchuk PJ. Tachycardia with pulses: narrow and wide. In: Field JM, Kudenchuk PJ, O'Connor RE, et al, editors. The textbook of emergency cardiovascular care and CPR. Philadelphia: Lippincott Williams & Wilkins; 2009. p. 313–40.
51. Goldenberg IF, Lewis WR, Dias VC, et al. Intravenous diltiazem for the treatment of patients with atrial fibrillation or flutter and moderate to severe congestive heart failure. Am J Cardiol 1994;74:884–9.
52. Gould LA, Betzu R, Vacek T, et al. Magnesium treatment of torsade de pointes—a case report. Angiology 1990;41:577–81.
53. Tzivoni D, Banai S, Schuger C, et al. Treatment of torsade de pointes with magnesium sulfate. Circulation 1988;77:392–7.
54. Winters SL, Sachs RG, Curwin JH. Nonsustained polymorphous ventricular tachycardia during amiodarone therapy for atrial fibrillation complicating cardiomyopathy. Management with intravenous magnesium sulfate. Chest 1997;111: 1454–7.
55. Pellegrini CN, Scheinman MM. Clinical management of ventricular tachycardia. Curr Probl Cardiol 2010;35:453–504.
56. Keren A, Tzivoni D, Gavish D, et al. Etiology, warning signs and therapy of torsade de pointes. A study of 10 patients. Circulation 1981;64:1167–74.
57. Goldberger ZD, Rho RW, Page RL. Approach to the diagnosis and initial management of the stable adult patient with a wide complex tachycardia. Am J Cardiol 2008;101:1456–66.
58. Marill KA, Wolfram S, Desouza IS, et al. Adenosine for wide-complex tachycardia: efficacy and safety. Crit Care Med 2009;37:2512–8.

59. Wilber DJ, Baerman JM, Olshansky B, et al. Adenosine-sensitive ventricular tachycardia. Clinical characteristics and response to catheter ablation. Circulation 1993;87:126–34.
60. Griffith MJ, Garratt CJ, Mounsey P, et al. Ventricular tachycardia as default diagnosis in broad complex tachycardia. Lancet 1994;343:386–8.
61. Callans DJ, Marchlinski FE. Dissociation of termination and prevention of inducibility of sustained ventricular tachycardia with infusion of procainamide: evidence for distinct mechanisms. J Am Coll Cardiol 1992;19:111–7.
62. Sharma AD, Purves P, Yee R, et al. Hemodynamic effects of intravenous procainamide during ventricular tachycardia. Am Heart J 1990;119:1034–41.
63. Marill KA, Desouza IS, Nishijima DK, et al. Amiodarone or procainamide for the termination of sustained stable ventricular tachycardia: an historical multicenter comparison. Acad Emerg Med 2010;17:297–306.
64. Ochi RP, Goldenberg IF, Almquist A, et al. Intravenous amiodarone for the rapid treatment of life-threatening ventricular arrhythmias in critically ill patients with coronary artery disease. Am J Cardiol 1989;64:599–603.
65. Somberg JC, Bailin SJ, Haffajee CI, et al. Intravenous lidocaine versus intravenous amiodarone (in a new aqueous formulation) for incessant ventricular tachycardia. Am J Cardiol 2002;90:853–9.
66. Marill KA, Desouza IS, Nishijima DK, et al. Amiodarone is poorly effective for the acute termination of ventricular tachycardia. Ann Emerg Med 2006;47:217–24.
67. Tomlinson DR, Cherian P, Betts TR, et al. Intravenous amiodarone for the pharmacological termination of haemodynamically-tolerated sustained ventricular tachycardia: is bolus dose amiodarone an appropriate first-line treatment? Emerg Med J 2008;25:15–8.
68. Levine JH, Massumi A, Scheinman MM, et al. Intravenous amiodarone for recurrent sustained hypotensive ventricular tachyarrhythmias. Intravenous Amiodarone Multicenter Trial Group. J Am Coll Cardiol 1996;27:67–75.
69. Somberg JC, Timar S, Bailin SJ, et al. Lack of a hypotensive effect with rapid administration of a new aqueous formulation of intravenous amiodarone. Am J Cardiol 2004;93:576–81.
70. Ho DS, Zecchin RP, Cooper MJ, et al. Rapid intravenous infusion of d-1 sotalol: time to onset of effects on ventricular refractoriness, and safety. Eur Heart J 1995;16:81–6.
71. Ho DS, Zecchin RP, Richards DA, et al. Double-blind trial of lignocaine versus sotalol for acute termination of spontaneous sustained ventricular tachycardia. Lancet 1994;344:18–23.
72. Wang YS, Scheinman MM, Chien WW, et al. Patients with supraventricular tachycardia presenting with aborted sudden death: incidence, mechanism and long-term follow-up. J Am Coll Cardiol 1991;18:1711–9.
73. Kim RJ, Gerling BR, Kono AT, et al. Precipitation of ventricular fibrillation by intravenous diltiazem and metoprolol in a young patient with occult Wolff-Parkinson-White syndrome. Pacing Clin Electrophysiol 2008;31:776–9.
74. Strasberg B, Sagie A, Rechavia E, et al. Deleterious effects of intravenous verapamil in Wolff-Parkinson-White patients and atrial fibrillation. Cardiovasc Drugs Ther 1989;2:801–6.
75. Li P. Electrophysiological properties of atrial fibrillation with WPW syndrome and the role of procainamide in conversion. Zhonghua Xin Xue Guan Bing Za Zhi 1991;19:65–6, 123 [in Chinese].
76. Schatz I, Ordog GJ, Karody R, et al. Wolff-Parkinson-White syndrome presenting in atrial fibrillation. Ann Emerg Med 1987;16:574–8.

77. Simonian SM, Lotfipour S, Wall C, et al. Challenging the superiority of amiodarone for rate control in Wolff-Parkinson-White and atrial fibrillation. Intern Emerg Med 2010;5:421–6.
78. Tijunelis MA, Herbert ME. Myth: intravenous amiodarone is safe in patients with atrial fibrillation and Wolff-Parkinson-White syndrome in the emergency department. CJEM 2005;7:262–5.
79. Fengler BT, Brady WJ, Plautz CU. Atrial fibrillation in the Wolff-Parkinson-White syndrome: ECG recognition and treatment in the ED. Am J Emerg Med 2007; 25:576–83.
80. Schützenberger W, Leisch F, Gmeiner R. Enhanced accessory pathway conduction following intravenous amiodarone in atrial fibrillation. A case report. Int J Cardiol 1987;16:93–5.
81. Kappenberger LJ, Fromer MA, Steinbrunn W, et al. Efficacy of amiodarone in the Wolff-Parkinson-White syndrome with rapid ventricular response via accessory pathway during atrial fibrillation. Am J Cardiol 1984;54:330–5.

Atrial Fibrillation

Laura J. Bontempo, MD[a],*, Eric Goralnick, MD[b]

KEYWORDS

• Atrial fibrillation • Atrial flutter • Heart • Dysrhythmia

OVERVIEW

Atrial fibrillation (AF) results from the chaotic depolarization of atrial tissue and is the most common dysrhythmia diagnosed in United States (US) emergency departments (EDs).[1] AF affects greater than 1% of the general population, with a peak prevalence of 10% in those greater than 80 years of age.[2,3] By 2050, it is estimated that nearly 16 million US patients will suffer from AF.[4] AF-related complaints accounted for an increase in ED visits of 88% between 1993 and 2003.[1]

AF is an independent risk factor for stroke, congestive heart failure, and overall mortality.[5] Rates of ischemic stroke in nonvalvular AF average 5% annually, 2 to 7 times the rate of the patient population without AF.[6] Overall mortality in patients with AF is almost double that of patients in normal sinus rhythm.[7]

AF not only has a significant health impact but it places a formidable economic burden on our health care system, accounting for $6.65 billion annually in direct and indirect costs.[8]

Emergency Medicine physicians are often tasked with management of new-onset or permanent AF. AF is termed paroxysmal when it terminates spontaneously in fewer than 7 days, and persistent when it is present beyond 7 days and requires cardioversion (electrical or pharmacologic) to terminate. Permanent AF is persistent AF for which cardioversion has failed or has not been attempted. Management strategies have traditionally encompassed rate control, rhythm control, and anticoagulation, but a lack of solid evidence has led to wide variations in ED physician practice.[9]

The recommendations in this article are derived from a combination of existing guidelines, additional evidence, and consensus.

CAUSES

It is imperative for the Emergency Medicine physician to identify and treat the serious and reversible underlying causes of AF.

[a] Department of Emergency Medicine, Yale University, 464 Congress Avenue, New Haven, CT 06519, USA
[b] Department of Emergency Medicine, Brigham and Women's Hospital and Harvard Medical School, 75 Francis Street, Neville House, Boston, MA 02115, USA
* Corresponding author.
E-mail address: laura.bontempo@yale.edu

Emerg Med Clin N Am 29 (2011) 747–758
doi:10.1016/j.emc.2011.08.008   emed.theclinics.com
0733-8627/11/$ – see front matter © 2011 Elsevier Inc. All rights reserved.

AF is most commonly associated with cardiovascular disease. Hypertension, coronary artery disease, cardiomyopathy, valvular disease, myocarditis, and pericarditis are the most common associations. AF may also occur after cardiac surgery. AF may result from another supraventricular tachycardia, in particular Wolff-Parkinson White, in which rapid hemodynamic collapse may occur as a result of accessory pathway conduction.

Hyperthyroidism, hypokalemia, sympathomimetic use, electrocution, and pulmonary disorders, including pulmonary embolism, are all noncardiac causes of AF. Excessive alcohol intake, termed holiday heart syndrome, is another noncardiac cause of AF and typically occurs after an alcohol binge in someone who is not accustomed to drinking large volumes of alcohol.

AF in patients less than age 60 years with no underlying cardiovascular disease is termed lone atrial fibrillation. It is particularly common in patients with paroxysmal AF, in which up to 45% of patients have no underlying cardiac disease identified.[10]

DIAGNOSIS

The uncoordinated activity of the atria results in irregular passage of impulses through the atrioventricular (AV) node to the ventricle. The patient may experience palpitations caused by the irregular, and often rapid, ventricular contractions. On examination, the clinician finds an irregular, likely tachycardic, pulse.

The electrocardiogram of a patient in AF does not have discernable, independent p-waves. Instead, the p-waves are replaced by fibrillatory waves that are rapid oscillations that vary in shape and amplitude. Because of the irregular conduction of these atrial fibrillatory impulses to the ventricles, QRS complexes occur with varying R-R intervals. Overall, this results in a rapid, narrow complex, irregular rhythm without discernable p-waves (**Fig. 1**).

If the atrial impulses conduct to the ventricle via an accessory pathway or if the impulse is interrupted by a ventricular conduction block (right or left bundle), the QRS complex will be wide. A sustained, rapid, irregular, wide complex tachycardia suggests AF with a bundle branch block or AF with conduction over an accessory pathway.

MANAGEMENT

When managing a patient with AF, the clinician must choose a strategy of rate control or rhythm control. Rhythm control is a strategy to terminate the AF and return the patient to normal sinus rhythm. A rate control strategy focuses on maintaining AF but at a controlled ventricular rate. The selected management strategy is primarily dependent on patient stability, severity of symptoms, duration of symptoms, and clinician preference.

The Atrial Fibrillation Follow-up Investigation of Rhythm Management (AFFIRM) study[11] and the Rate Control versus Electrical Cardioversion for Persistent Atrial Fibrillation (RACE) study[12] compared the outcomes of patients treated with a rate versus rhythm control strategy and found no significant difference in survival or

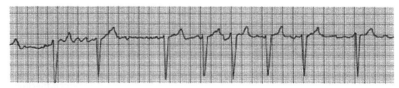

Fig. 1. Atrial fibrillation.

quality-of-life advantage between the 2 groups.[13] The AFFIRM study enrolled more than 4000 patients and the RACE study enrolled more than 500 patients. Both studies examined issues of morbidity and mortality in patients with AF treated with rate and rhythm control. Higher rates of thromboembolic events were seen in the rhythm control group in both studies; however, these events occurred in patients who were not adequately anticoagulated.[12,13]

When using either strategy for the management of AF, the patient's thromboembolic risk must be evaluated and therapy for prevention of thromboembolism must be initiated, as appropriate. The risk of a thromboembolic stroke when using a rhythm control strategy is equal to that of rate control plus anticoagulation.[14]

For patients with AF in whom the duration of the AF is unknown or known to be greater than 48 hours, a rate control strategy is preferred until adequate anticoagulation is achieved or an intracardiac thrombus is ruled out through an echocardiogram. In any patient with hemodynamic instability caused by their AF, the dysrhythmia must be terminated and, therefore, a rhythm control strategy is necessary.

RATE CONTROL

The goal of a rate control strategy for AF is to control the ventricular rate of the dysrhythmia without terminating the AF.

The American College of Cardiology (ACC), The American Heart Association (AHA), and the European Society of Cardiology (ESC), in their 2006 guidelines, recommend a resting heart rate of 60 to 80 beats per minute and a moderate exercise heart rate of 90 to 115 beats per minute as an adequate endpoint for patients with rate-controlled atrial fibrillation.[14] However, new data challenge the need for strict heart rate control and propose a more lenient rate control of a resting heart rate less than 110 beats per minute.[15] The comparison of the strict versus lenient approaches showed similar patient outcomes and no significant difference in the prevalence of AF symptoms for patients with a left ventricular ejection fraction greater than 40%.[16] Lenient heart rate control parameters may be easier to achieve in the ED and maintain as an outpatient, thereby making rate control a simpler option for patients and health care providers.[15] In follow-up, a patient's heart rate can be checked during visits to health care providers or via a 24-hour ambulatory electrocardiogram monitor.

Rate control is mainly accomplished by using agents that prolong the refractory period of the AV node. The 2 main classes of medications used are β-blockers and calcium channel antagonists. Digoxin may be used as an adjust agent but, because of its delayed therapeutic onset, its emergent usefulness is limited. Both β-blockers and calcium channel antagonists are effective in obtaining rate control. However, in the AFFIRM trial, β-blockers were found to achieve strict heart rate control in 70% of patients versus 54% of patients when calcium channel antagonists were used.[13] In light of the new data suggesting that lenient heart rate control is equally beneficial to strict heart rate control, the benefit of β-blockers versus calcium channel antagonists as rate controlling agents must be reexamined. In the ED, rate control of AF with rapid ventricular response may be accomplished via intravenous administration of either class of medications.

Commonly used β-blockers are metoprolol, esmolol, and propranolol. The possible side effects of these drugs include hypotension, heart block, bradycardia, bronchospasm, and heart failure.[14] Therefore, β-blockers should be used cautiously in patients with AF and hypotension or heart failure from a depressed ejection fraction.[14]

Commonly used calcium channel antagonists are diltiazem and verapamil. Both drugs have similar safety profiles, including their effects on blood pressure.[17]

Diltiazem is classically dosed at 0.25 mg/kg intravenously (IV) in 2 minutes, although doses less than 0.2 mg/kg have been shown to be effective with a decreased risk of hypotension.[18] In addition to hypotension, the possible side effects of calcium channel antagonists are heart block and heart failure. Calcium channel antagonists do not have the side effect of bronchospasm and, therefore, may be preferred in patients with chronic obstructive pulmonary disease or asthma.

Digoxin works by enhancing vagal activity on the AV node and increasing its refractory period. This action, in turn, decreases the ventricular rate. The onset of action for intravenous digoxin is at least 60 minutes and its peak effect can take up to 6 hours.[14] These pharmacokinetics make digoxin of limited usefulness in the acute management of AF with a rapid ventricular response. However, digoxin does lower resting heart rates in patients with AF and is best used as an adjunct in patients treated with a β-blocker or calcium channel antagonist.[19] Digoxin does not slow the heart rate during exercise in patients with AF.

Once rate control is obtained, the patient must be transitioned to the oral equivalent of whichever agent achieved the rate control **Table 1**.

RHYTHM CONTROL

The goal of a rhythm control strategy is to terminate the AF and restore and maintain sinus rhythm.

A critical piece of information for any emergency physician contemplating a rate control strategy is the duration of the patient's AF. The risk of a thromboembolic event increases when the duration of the AF exceeds 48 hours. If the duration of the AF is greater than 48 hours or is unknown, a rhythm control strategy should not be pursued from the ED. Instead, the ventricular response rate should be controlled (as discussed earlier) and anticoagulation initiated.

The 2 main modes of rhythm control are pharmacologic cardioversion and electrical cardioversion. The risk of a thromboembolic event is the same with pharmacologic and electrical cardioversion and, therefore, the guidelines for anticoagulation are the same for both methods.[14]

Direct current electrical cardioversion (DCCV) can be attempted with a synchronized monophasic shock or a synchronized biphasic shock. Biphasic shocks have a higher success rate for restoration of sinus rhythm and success is achieved using fewer

Table 1 Rate control agents		
Medication	**IV Loading Dose**	**Oral Dose**
β-Blockers		
Esmolol	500 μg/kg then 60 μg/kg/min	Not available
Metoprolol	5 mg every 5 min, 3 dose maximum	25–100 mg twice daily
Propranolol	0.15 mg/kg	80–240 mg daily in divided doses
Calcium Channel Antagonists		
Diltiazem	0.25 mg/kg then 5–15 mg/h	120–360 mg daily in divided doses or slow-release form
Verapamil	0.075–0.15 mg/kg	240–360 mg daily, divided doses or slow-release form
Digoxin	0.25–0.5 mg	0.125–0.375 mg daily

joules. In a head-to-head study comparing the efficacy of monophasic shocks with biphasic shocks in AF, biphasic shocks had a success rate of 94% whereas the monophasic shock had a success rate of 79%.[20] Biphasic shock waveforms are, therefore, the standard of care for DCCV of AF.[14]

The overall success rate of DCCV is 70% to 90%.[21,22] Predictors for successful cardioversion include shorter duration of AF, younger age, and lower thoracic impedance.[14,22] DCCV is less likely to be successful in patients with left atrial enlargement, underlying heart disease, and cardiomegaly.[22] The rate of recurrence of AF after cardioversion is high, with one study finding that only 23% of patients remained in sinus rhythm 1 year after successful cardioversion.[23] However, DCCV, is a low-risk procedure and does not incur the risk of adverse drug effects seen with pharmacologic agents. If time permits, patients should be procedurally sedated before DCCV.

Pretreating a patient with the antidysrhythmic ibutilide (1 mg infused in 10 minutes then waiting 10 minutes before DCCV), facilitates successful cardioversion. This pretreatment has also been shown to reduce the number of DCCV attempts and the amount of energy required for biphasic cardioversion.[24]

Pharmacologic attempts at cardioversion are less effective than DCCV using a biphasic waveform[14]; nonetheless, many agents are available for pharmacologic cardioversion. Of the options available, 4 agents have class I, level of evidence A recommendations from the ACC, AHA, and ESC. These are: flecainide, propafenone, ibutilide, and dofetilide (**Table 2**).[14]

Flecainide is a Vaughan Williams class Ic antiarrhythmic that acts through sodium channel inhibition. Flecainide can be given intravenously or orally and is more effective than amiodarone, propafenone, and placebo in converting AF to sinus rhythm.[25–28] After a single oral dose, 75% to 91% of patients with AF convert within 8 hours.[29] Flecainide should not be used for patients with a history of acute coronary ischemia, structural heart disease, or cardiomyopathy.[30]

Propafenone is also a class Ic antiarrhythmic that can be given orally or intravenously. Oral propafenone has a cardioversion rate between 56% and 83% within 6

Table 2
Agents for pharmacologic cardioversion that have class I or class II, level of evidence A recommendations

Drug	AF Conversion Dose	Maintenance Dose	Comments
Flecainide	200 mg orally, or 2 mg/kg IV in 10 min	100 mg twice a day	May repeat oral dose if needed after 4 h Avoid in patients with history of ACS, structural heart disease, or cardiomyopathy
Propafenone	600 mg orally, or 2 mg/kg IV in 10 min	150–300 mg three times a day	Avoid in patients with history of ACS, structural heart disease, or cardiomyopathy
Ibutilide	1 mg IV in 10 min; may repeat once	—	Risk of torsades de pointes
Amiodarone	6 mg/kg IV in 60 min then 1.2 g in 24 h	600 mg daily for 1 month then taper	Slow onset Risk of hypotension

Abbreviation: ACS, acute coronary syndrome.

hours of administration. Intravenous propafenone has a shorter onset of action and results in more cardioversions within the first 2 hours.[14] Its safety profile is good, with significant adverse side effects being uncommon.[31] The use of propafenone should be avoided in patients with structural heart disease, heart failure and severe obstructive lung disease.[14]

Ibutilide is a class III antiarrhythmic that acts as a potassium channel blocker and prolongs the refractory period of the atrial and ventricular myocardium, the accessory pathway, and the AV node.[31] It is given as a single intravenous dose that may be repeated once if necessary. It has a conversion rate of 75% in recent-onset AF. For patients with atrial flutter, the conversion rate is greater than 80% by 30 minutes after administration.[32]

The main serious side effect of ibutilide is QT interval lengthening and subsequent ventricular dysrhythmias. There is a 4% risk of torsades de pointes and a 5% risk of monomorphic ventricular tachycardia. Patients at higher risk for torsades de pointes are those with small body size, a history of heart failure, nonwhite race, and women.[33] In addition, caution should be used for patients with ischemia, heart failure, and prior myocardial infarction, because torsades de pointes can be refractory to treatment in these patients.

Most episodes of ibutilide-induced torsades de pointes occur within 1 hour after treatment and almost all occur within 6 hours. Because of these dysrhythmia risks, patients must be monitored between 4 and 6 hours after drug administration. The risk of both torsades de pointes and ventricular tachycardia can be reduced by pre-treating with 4 g of magnesium. This pretreatment also improves the efficacy of ibutilide for cardioversion of AF.[34] Hypokalemia should also be corrected before ibutilide treatment.

Dofetilide is a class III antiarrhythmic. It is primarily used for patients with persistent AF and, therefore, is of limited use to the emergency physician. Because of its complex dosing and potential to induce malignant dysrhythmias, once administered, patients require 72 hours of in-hospital monitoring.[35] Dofetilide has been studied in multiple large trials and is a moderately effective agent for pharmacocardioversion of patients with persistent AF.

In addition to these agents, procainamide may be considered. Procainamide has an ACC/AHA/ESC class IIb recommendation, with level of evidence B[14]; however, it was the agent used to attempt pharmacologic cardioversion in the Ottawa Aggressive Protocol (OAP). In this protocol, procainamide resulted in conversion to sinus rhythm for 59.9% of patients in AF and 28.1% of patients in atrial flutter.[36]

The OAP deserves special attention because it sequentially combines the use of pharmacocardioversion and DCCV for patients with recent-onset AF or atrial flutter.

In this protocol, patients who presented to the Ottawa Hospital ED with recent-onset AF or atrial flutter were treated with a rhythm control strategy. Recent-onset AF or flutter were defined as symptoms clearly present for fewer than 48 hours unless the patient was already therapeutically anticoagulated with warfarin for 3 weeks. Stable patients received procainamide 1 g infused in 1 hour. If procainamide failed to convert the patient to sinus rhythm, or if pharmacologic cardioversion was not attempted (because of physician choice), DCCV was performed. DCCV was successful for 91% of patients in AF and 100% of patients in atrial flutter. The adverse event rate was low for all OAP patients, with the most common adverse event being transient hypotension.[36]

The OAP successfully showed the feasibility of a rhythm control strategy in the ED. Overall, 96.8% of the enrolled patients were discharged to home, with 93.3% leaving in sinus rhythm. The overall average ED length of stay for enrolled patients was

4.9 hours. Follow-up was conducted for 7 days after the index ED visit and, within this time, 8.6% of patients had a relapse of their AF. Patients who are rhythm controlled in the ED must, therefore, have close follow-up arranged and consideration should be given to oral antiarrhythmic drugs for rhythm maintenance.

ANTICOAGULATION

AF is the most common cause of cardioembolic stroke and confers increased morbidity and mortality compared with non-AF stroke.[37] Effective antithrombotic therapy is both a critical and controversial component of AF management.

The $CHADS_2$ (chronic heart failure, hypertension, advanced age, diabetes, and stroke/transient ischemic attack) scoring system was derived to predict cardioembolic stroke risk based on risk factors in patients with nonanticoagulated, nonvalvular AF and to guide antithrombotic therapy.[38] In this scoring system, 1 point is assigned for chronic heart failure, hypertension, advanced age, and diabetes, and 2 points for prior stroke/transient ischemic attack (**Table 3**).

The stroke rate per 100 patient years without antithrombotic therapy increased by a factor of 1.5 for each point in the $CHADS_2$ score. Patients with a score of 0 are low risk and may be managed solely with aspirin 325 mg daily. Moderate-risk patients are those with a score of 1 and anticoagulation with vitamin K antagonist (VKA) versus aspirin is based on a clinician's discretion. High-risk patients, with a score of 2 or greater, should be treated with VKA in the absence of contraindications.

The risk and difficulty of maintaining some patients on oral anticoagulation has prompted investigation into alternative treatments. The Atrial Fibrillation Clopidogrel Trial with Irbesartan for Prevention of Vascular Events (ACTIVE-W) trial compared clopidogrel plus aspirin with warfarin therapy for the prevention of vascular events in moderate-risk and high-risk patients with AF. Warfarin was found to be superior for the prevention of vascular events without having a higher risk of bleeding events.[39]

The Effect of Clopidogrel Added to Aspirin in Patients with Atrial Fibrillation (ACTIVE-A) study compared clopidogrel and aspirin with aspirin-only treatment in patients deemed unsuitable for oral anticoagulation therapy.[40] This study found that the combination of clopidogrel plus aspirin reduced the risk of major vascular events but increased the risk of major hemorrhage.

Table 3 CHADS₂ score		
CHADS₂ Score	**95% CI**	**Yearly Risk of Stroke (%)**
0	1.2–3.0	1.9
1	2.0–3.8	2.8
2	3.1–5.1	4
3	4.6–7.3	5.9
4	6.3–11.1	8.5
5	8.2–17.5	12.5
6	10.5–27.4	18.2

Abbreviation: CI, confidence interval.

Yearly risk of stroke in patients with AF without antithrombotic therapy. Prior stroke, 2 points; congestive heart failure, 1 point; hypertension, 1 point; diabetes, 1 point; age 75 years or older, 1 point.

Predominately based on these 2 studies, the AHA, the ACC Foundation, and the Heart Rhythm Society in 2011 jointly recommend considering the use of clopidogrel plus aspirin in patients with AF in whom oral anticoagulation is unsuitable because of "patient preference or the physician's assessment of the patient's ability to safely sustain anticoagulation."[16]

There is an increased risk of thromboembolism and stroke in patients in AF for greater than 48 hours.[41] The incidence of thromboembolism or stroke in patients with AF of duration less than 48 hours is less than 1%.[42] Hemodynamically stable patients with AF duration of less than 48 hours can undergo cardioversion and do not require anticoagulation before the procedure. Patients with an AF duration of greater than 48 hours should receive anticoagulation for 3 weeks before and 4 weeks after cardioversion. Patients who undergo transesophageal echocardiography with no evidence of left atrial thrombus should continue anticoagulation for 4 weeks after the cardioversion procedure. Those with thrombus should use anticoagulation for 3 weeks and repeat the transesophageal echocardiography to ensure thrombus resolution before cardioversion.[43] These guidelines apply to patients undergoing both pharmacologic and electrical cardioversion.

VKAs AND ASPIRIN

VKA therapy is recommended in patients with a CHADS$_2$ score of 2 points or higher. For patients with a CHADS$_2$ score of 1, VKA may be recommended over aspirin if thromboembolic risk is higher than the risk of bleeding complications.

VKA and aspirin, the only antithrombotic therapies approved by the American College of Chest Physicians, reduce the risk of ischemic stroke by 64% and 22%, respectively.[44,45] However, VKA therapy requires regular monitoring, has labile drug and food interactions, pharmacogenetic variability, and significant risk of major bleeding. VKA also has a narrow therapeutic window. A goal international normalized ratio (INR) of 2 to 3 is only achieved two-thirds of the time in randomized controlled trials and even less in clinical practice.[46] Because of these limitations, VKAs are only prescribed in two-thirds of patients with AF.[47]

HEPARIN AND LOW-MOLECULAR-WEIGHT HEPARIN

Unfractionated heparin (UFH) and low-molecular-weight heparin (LMWH) act by binding to antithrombin and inhibiting both thrombin and activated factor Xa.

A randomized control trial compared an initial antithrombotic regime of tinzaparin (a LMWH) with conventional intravenous UFH in 96 patients with new-onset, acute AF who initially presented to an ED. Five patients in the UFH group compared with zero patients in the LMWH group developed ischemic stroke/transient ischemic attack during the first 48 hours.[48]

The AHA, ACC, and ESC do not offer any guidelines for the use of UFH versus LMWH.[14]

DIRECT THROMBIN INHIBITORS

Because of difficulties with warfarin therapy, various novel anticoagulant drugs are currently undergoing trials to find an oral medication that does not require frequent monitoring and can be administered at a fixed dose.

Both the intrinsic coagulation pathway (involving factors XII, XI, IX, and VIII) and the extrinsic coagulation pathway (involving factor VII) end in the same common pathway, the activation of factor X to factor Xa. Factor Xa, along with factor Va, activates prothrombin (factor II) to thrombin (factor IIa). Thrombin not only activates fibrinogen into fibrin (factor Ia) but also activates factors V, VII, VIII, IX, and XIII. Novel orally available inhibitors directly inhibit factor Xa or factor IIa, hence blocking thrombin and inhibiting coagulation.

Dabigatran is the most promising (and only) oral direct thrombin inhibitor with data from a phase III trial for stroke prevention in patients with AF. The RE-LY (Randomized Evaluation of Long-term Anticoagulation Therapy) trial included 18,113 patients with AF. Stroke or systemic embolism occurred as often in those patients taking 100 mg of dabigatran twice daily as in those taking warfarin (1.5% vs 1.7%). The incidence of hemorrhagic stroke and all-cause mortality were both reduced in the patients on dabigatran.[49] However, patients on dabigatran had increased incidence of gastrointestinal bleeding and myocardial infarction.[49] Dabigatran is nonreversible and this must also be considered when evaluating its risk/benefit ratio for a patient.

ATRIAL FLUTTER

Atrial flutter is, electrophysiologically, a separate entity from AF; however, most of the management guidelines discussed earlier also apply to this disease entity. The emergency medicine and cardiology literature cited earlier has similar recommendations for rate control, rhythm control, and anticoagulation in either AF or atrial flutter.[50–52]

However, atrial flutter is difficult to rate control and therefore a rhythm control strategy may be necessary. Ibutilide is the agent of choice for pharmacologic rhythm control with atrial flutter; however, DCCV may be necessary for a sustained return to sinus rhythm. In a retrospective cohort study of 122 patients at 2 urban EDs, patients in atrial flutter undergoing DCCV successfully achieved normal sinus rhythm 91% of the time, and those undergoing antiarrhythmic pharmacocardioversion achieved sinus rhythm 27% of the time. Of those patients electrically cardioverted, 17% required greater than 150 J for successful electrocardioversion to sinus rhythm. Although 3 patients died within the 1 year follow-up time frame, no patients suffered a stroke.[53]

DISPOSITION

After rate or rhythm control is accomplished, underlying inciting events are addressed, anticoagulation is initiated, and close follow-up is established, patients with new-onset AF may be considered for discharge from the ED. Discharged patients should be symptom free or symptom controlled, hemodynamically stable, and without evidence of myocardial ischemia or other serious cause of their AF. The Canadian Cardiovascular Society recommends admission for highly symptomatic patients with decompensated heart failure, myocardial ischemia, or inadequate rate control.[48]

Follow-up is essential to identify potential underlying structural heart disease, to monitor heart rate, and rhythm, and to ensure adequate anticoagulation, such as INR monitoring. The duration of antiarrhythmic and anticoagulation therapy, as well as the necessity of cardiac imaging, also need to be addressed in follow-up.

REFERENCES

1. McDonald AJ, Pelletier AJ, Ellinor PT, et al. Increasing US emergency department visit rates and subsequent hospital admissions for atrial fibrillation from 1993 to 2004. Ann Emerg Med 2008;51:58–65.
2. Go AS, Hylek EM, Phillips KA, et al. Prevalence of diagnosed atrial fibrillation in adults: national implications for rhythm management and stroke prevention: the

AnTicoagulation and Risk Factors in Atrial Fibrillation (ATRIA) Study. JAMA 2001; 285:2370–5.

3. Feinberg WM, Blackshear JL, Laupacis A, et al. Prevalence, age distribution, and gender of patients with atrial fibrillation. Analysis and implications. Arch Intern Med 1995;155:469–73.

4. Miyasaka Y, Barnes ME, Gersh BJ, et al. Secular trends in incidence of atrial fibrillation in Olmsted County, Minnesota, 1980 to 2000, and implications on the projections for future prevalence. Circulation 2006;114:119–25.

5. Stewart S, Hart CL, Hole DJ, et al. A population-based study of the long-term risks associated with atrial fibrillation: 20-year follow-up of the Renfrew/Paisley study. Am J Med 2002;113:359–64.

6. Wolf PA, Abbott RD, Kannel WB. Atrial fibrillation as an independent risk factor for stroke: the Framingham Study. Stroke 1991;22:983–8.

7. Krahn AD, Manfreda J, Tate RB, et al. The natural history of atrial fibrillation: incidence, risk factors, and prognosis in the Manitoba Follow-Up Study. Am J Med 1995;98:476–84.

8. Coyne KS, Paramore C, Grandy S, et al. Assessing the direct costs of treating nonvalvular atrial fibrillation in the United States. Value Health 2006;9:348–56.

9. Stiell IG, Clement CM, Brison RJ, et al. Variation in management of recent-onset atrial fibrillation and flutter among academic hospital emergency departments. Ann Emerg Med 2011;57:13–21.

10. Page RL. Clinical practice. Newly diagnosed atrial fibrillation. N Engl J Med 2004; 351:2408–16.

11. Curtis AB, Gersh BJ, Corley SD, et al. Clinical factors that influence response to treatment strategies in atrial fibrillation: the Atrial Fibrillation Follow-up Investigation of Rhythm Management (AFFIRM) study. Am Heart J 2005;149:645–9.

12. Van Gelder IC, Hagens VE, Bosker HA, et al. A comparison of rate control and rhythm control in patients with recurrent persistent atrial fibrillation. N Engl J Med 2002;347:1834–40.

13. Wyse DG, Waldo AL, DiMarco JP, et al. A comparison of rate control and rhythm control in patients with atrial fibrillation. N Engl J Med 2002;347:1825–33.

14. Fuster V, Ryden LE, Cannom DS, et al. ACC/AHA/ESC 2006 Guidelines for the Management of Patients with Atrial Fibrillation: a report of the American College of Cardiology/American Heart Association Task Force on Practice Guidelines and the European Society of Cardiology Committee for Practice Guidelines (Writing Committee to Revise the 2001 Guidelines for the Management of Patients With Atrial Fibrillation): developed in collaboration with the European Heart Rhythm Association and the Heart Rhythm Society. Circulation 2006;114:e257–354.

15. Van Gelder IC, Groenveld HF, Crijns HJ, et al. Lenient versus strict rate control in patients with atrial fibrillation. N Engl J Med 2010;362:1363–73.

16. Wann LS, Curtis AB, January CT, et al. 2011 ACCF/AHA/HRS focused update on the management of patients with atrial fibrillation (updating the 2006 guideline): a report of the American College of Cardiology Foundation/American Heart Association Task Force on Practice Guidelines. Circulation 2011;123:104–23.

17. Phillips BG, Gandhi AJ, Sanoski CA, et al. Comparison of intravenous diltiazem and verapamil for the acute treatment of atrial fibrillation and atrial flutter. Pharmacotherapy 1997;17:1238–45.

18. Lee J, Kim K, Lee CC, et al. Low-dose diltiazem in atrial fibrillation with rapid ventricular response. Am J Emerg Med 2010. [Epub ahead of print].

19. Tamariz LJ, Bass EB. Pharmacological rate control of atrial fibrillation. Cardiol Clin 2004;22:35–45.

20. Mittal S, Ayati S, Stein KM, et al. Transthoracic cardioversion of atrial fibrillation: comparison of rectilinear biphasic versus damped sine wave monophasic shocks. Circulation 2000;101:1282–7.
21. Gowda SA, Shah A, Steinberg JS. Cardioversion of atrial fibrillation. Prog Cardiovasc Dis 2005;48:88–107.
22. Van Gelder IC, Crijns HJ, Van Gilst WH, et al. Prediction of uneventful cardioversion and maintenance of sinus rhythm from direct-current electrical cardioversion of chronic atrial fibrillation and flutter. Am J Cardiol 1991;68:41–6.
23. Siaplaouras S, Jung J, Buob A, et al. Incidence and management of early recurrent atrial fibrillation (ERAF) after transthoracic electrical cardioversion. Europace 2004;6:15–20.
24. Mazzocca G, Corbucci G, Venturini E, et al. Is pretreatment with ibutilide useful for atrial fibrillation cardioversion when combined with biphasic shock? J Cardiovasc Med (Hagerstown) 2006;7:124–8.
25. Donovan KD, Power BM, Hockings BE, et al. Intravenous flecainide versus amiodarone for recent-onset atrial fibrillation. Am J Cardiol 1995;75:693–7.
26. Donovan KD, Dobb GJ, Coombs LJ, et al. Efficacy of flecainide for the reversion of acute onset atrial fibrillation. Am J Cardiol 1992;70:50A–4A [discussion: 54A–5A].
27. Martinez-Marcos FJ, Garcia-Garmendia JL, Ortega-Carpio A, et al. Comparison of intravenous flecainide, propafenone, and amiodarone for conversion of acute atrial fibrillation to sinus rhythm. Am J Cardiol 2000;86:950–3.
28. Capucci A, Lenzi T, Boriani G, et al. Effectiveness of loading oral flecainide for converting recent-onset atrial fibrillation to sinus rhythm in patients without organic heart disease or with only systemic hypertension. Am J Cardiol 1992;70:69–72.
29. Khan IA. Oral loading single dose flecainide for pharmacological cardioversion of recent-onset atrial fibrillation. Int J Cardiol 2003;87:121–8.
30. National Guideline C. Atrial fibrillation. National clinical guideline for management in primary and secondary care. Rockville (MD): Agency for Healthcare Research and Quality (AHRQ); 2006.
31. Glatter KA, Dorostkar PC, Yang Y, et al. Electrophysiological effects of ibutilide in patients with accessory pathways. Circulation 2001;104:1933–9.
32. Ando G, Di Rosa S, Rizzo F, et al. Ibutilide for cardioversion of atrial flutter: efficacy of a single dose in recent-onset arrhythmias. Minerva Cardioangiol 2004;52:37–42.
33. Gowda RM, Khan IA, Wilbur SL, et al. Torsade de pointes: the clinical considerations. Int J Cardiol 2004;96:1–6.
34. Steinwender C, Honig S, Kypta A, et al. Pre-injection of magnesium sulfate enhances the efficacy of ibutilide for the conversion of typical but not of atypical persistent atrial flutter. Int J Cardiol 2010;141:260–5.
35. Singh S, Zoble RG, Yellen L, et al. Efficacy and safety of oral dofetilide in converting to and maintaining sinus rhythm in patients with chronic atrial fibrillation or atrial flutter: the Symptomatic Atrial Fibrillation Investigative Research on Dofetilide (SAFIRE-D) study. Circulation 2000;102:2385–90.
36. Stiell IG, Clement CM, Perry JJ, et al. Association of the Ottawa Aggressive Protocol with rapid discharge of emergency department patients with recent-onset atrial fibrillation or flutter. CJEM 2010;12:181–91.
37. Marini C, De Santis F, Sacco S, et al. Contribution of atrial fibrillation to incidence and outcome of ischemic stroke: results from a population-based study. Stroke 2005;36:1115–9.
38. Gage BF, Waterman AD, Shannon W, et al. Validation of clinical classification schemes for predicting stroke: results from the National Registry of Atrial Fibrillation. JAMA 2001;285:2864–70.

39. Connolly S, Pogue J, Hart R, et al. Clopidogrel plus aspirin versus oral anticoagulation for atrial fibrillation in the Atrial fibrillation Clopidogrel Trial with Irbesartan for prevention of Vascular Events (ACTIVE W): a randomised controlled trial. Lancet 2006;367:1903–12.

40. Connolly SJ, Pogue J, Hart RG, et al. Effect of clopidogrel added to aspirin in patients with atrial fibrillation. N Engl J Med 2009;360:2066–78.

41. Raghavan AV, Decker WW, Meloy TD. Management of atrial fibrillation in the emergency department. Emerg Med Clin North Am 2005;23:1127–39.

42. Weigner MJ, Caulfield TA, Danias PG, et al. Risk for clinical thromboembolism associated with conversion to sinus rhythm in patients with atrial fibrillation lasting less than 48 hours. Ann Intern Med 1997;126:615–20.

43. Klein AL, Murray RD, Grimm RA. Role of transesophageal echocardiography-guided cardioversion of patients with atrial fibrillation. J Am Coll Cardiol 2001; 37:691–704.

44. Hart RG, Pearce LA, Aguilar MI. Meta-analysis: antithrombotic therapy to prevent stroke in patients who have nonvalvular atrial fibrillation. Ann Intern Med 2007; 146:857–67.

45. Ansell J, Hirsh J, Hylek E, et al. Pharmacology and management of the vitamin K antagonists: American College of Chest Physicians Evidence-Based Clinical Practice Guidelines (8th Edition). Chest 2008;133:160S–98S.

46. Matchar DB, Samsa GP, Cohen SJ, et al. Improving the quality of anticoagulation of patients with atrial fibrillation in managed care organizations: results of the managing anticoagulation services trial. Am J Med 2002;113:42–51.

47. Boulanger L, Kim J, Friedman M, et al. Patterns of use of antithrombotic therapy and quality of anticoagulation among patients with non-valvular atrial fibrillation in clinical practice. Int J Clin Pract 2006;60:258–64.

48. Siu CW, Jim MH, Lau CP, et al. Low molecular weight heparin versus unfractionated heparin for thromboprophylaxis in patients with acute atrial fibrillation: a randomized control trial. Acute Card Care 2011. [Epub ahead of print].

49. Wallentin L, Yusuf S, Ezekowitz MD, et al. Efficacy and safety of dabigatran compared with warfarin at different levels of international normalised ratio control for stroke prevention in atrial fibrillation: an analysis of the RE-LY trial. Lancet 2010;376:975–83.

50. Stiell IG, Clement CM, Symington C, et al. Emergency department use of intravenous procainamide for patients with acute atrial fibrillation or flutter. Acad Emerg Med 2007;14:1158–64.

51. Domanovits H, Schillinger M, Thoennissen J, et al. Termination of recent-onset atrial fibrillation/flutter in the emergency department: a sequential approach with intravenous ibutilide and external electrical cardioversion. Resuscitation 2000;45:181–7.

52. Fuster V, Rydén LE, Cannom DS, et al. ACC/AHA/ESC 2006 guidelines for the management of patients with atrial fibrillation: full text: a report of the American College of Cardiology/American Heart Association Task Force on practice guidelines and the European Society of Cardiology Committee for Practice Guidelines (Writing Committee to Revise the 2001 Guidelines for the Management of Patients with Atrial Fibrillation) developed in collaboration with the European Heart Rhythm Association and the Heart Rhythm Society. Europace 2006; 8:651–745.

53. Scheuermeyer FX, Grafstein E, Heilbron B, et al. Emergency department management and 1-year outcomes of patients with atrial flutter. Ann Emerg Med 2011;57:564.e2–71.e2.

Emergency Echocardiography

Anthony J. Weekes, MD[a,b,*], Dale P. Quirke, MD[c]

KEYWORDS

- Emergency echocardiography • Cardiac ultrasound
- Emergency medicine • Point-of-care cardiac ultrasound
- Focused cardiac ultrasound

CASE 1

Your next patient presents with a chief complaint of feeling "weak and dizzy." She has had gradual worsening shortness of breath for 2 weeks, a slight cough that is worse at night, and mild leg swelling. She denies any chest pain or fever. Her blood pressure is 88/58 mm Hg; heart rate is 120 beats per minute with a regular rhythm; respiratory rate is 28 breaths per minute with an oxygen saturation of 98% on room air; and her temperature is 99.3°F (37.4°C). Her physical examination is remarkable for distant heart sounds, bilateral rales at the lung bases, and moderate neck vein distention. Her abdomen is nontender and her legs are slightly edematous bilaterally. While the nurse inserts an intravenous line and draws tubes of blood, you bring in the ultrasound machine for a closer look.

SCOPE

The practice of emergency medicine has evolved to now include competence in emergency ultrasound as a basic training requirement of emergency medicine residency graduates. Over the past 10 years, advancements have been made in emergency ultrasound such that the use of ultrasound technology has now become integral to the daily practice of emergency medicine in the community as well as academic institutions. Emergency echocardiography (also referred to as "bedside cardiac ultrasound," "goal-directed cardiac ultrasound," "point-of-care cardiac ultrasound," "focused cardiac ultrasound" [FOCUS], or "bedside echo") is a well-established core application of emergency ultrasound. Emergency echocardiography that is

The authors have nothing to disclose.
[a] Department of Emergency Medicine, University of North Carolina, Chapel Hill, NC, USA
[b] Emergency Ultrasound Fellowship, Department of Emergency Medicine, Carolinas Medical Center, 1000 Blythe Boulevard, Charlotte, NC 28203, USA
[c] Bay Area Emergency Physicians, 611 South Fort Harrison, #354, Clearwater, FL 33756, USA
* Corresponding author. Emergency Ultrasound Fellowship, Department of Emergency Medicine, Carolinas Medical Center, 1000 Blythe Boulevard, Charlotte, NC 28203.
E-mail address: Anthony.Weekes@carolinashealthcare.org

performed and interpreted by emergency physicians is supported by the American College of Emergency Physicians (ACEP), the Society for Academic Emergency Medicine (SAEM), and the American Society of Echocardiography (ASE).[1,2,3] This article discusses the current indications, goals, and limitations of emergency transthoracic echocardiography. Training and quality assurance issues related to emergency echocardiography are not discussed in detail. For the majority of emergency physicians using emergency echocardiography, the main scope of practice is to evaluate for the presence or absence of a pericardial effusion, provide a visual estimation ("gestalt") of overall heart function and, to some extent, identify right heart strain and evaluate the inferior vena cava. Emergency ultrasound education is a requirement in the emergency medicine residency curriculum. Out of an increased presence of emergency ultrasound fellowships and the spread of emergency ultrasound education and programs to community emergency medicine practices, there is an emerging cadre of recently graduated and practicing emergency medicine and critical care physicians with an increased interest, level of use, and expertise in emergency echocardiography.[3,4,5]

Most of the discussion is centered on the uses, benefits, and limitations of clinically indicated emergency echocardiography as consulted by, if not performed by, the emergency physician.

EMERGENCY ECHOCARDIOGRAPHY IS GOAL-DIRECTED

Comprehensive echocardiography is traditionally performed by a certified echocardiographer in an echocardiography laboratory, and interpreted by a cardiologist. By contrast, emergency echocardiography attempts to answer a focused clinical question at the bedside in a time-sensitive manner. It is usually performed and interpreted by the treating physician. Emergency echocardiography is often indicated in the case of the patient who is overtly critically ill or in extremis. However, it can also help to rapidly unmask ominous underlying cardiac pathology in patients with otherwise deceptively mild symptoms. Information obtained can help to stratify cardiac function, identify structural abnormalities, or narrow the differential diagnosis of a patient presenting in shock. Goal-directed echocardiography, when immediately available to the treating physician, is a rapid, repeatable, and accurate test for diagnosing cardiac conditions critical to the care of the emergency department (ED) patient.

Echocardiography can be incorporated into the diagnostic and resuscitative phases of clinical care, as well as for safety in procedural guidance. The American College of Cardiology/American Heart Association Task Force on Practice Guidelines for the Clinical Application of Echocardiography includes common high-acuity situations seen daily in EDs. These indications include, but are not limited to, unexplained hypotension, dyspnea, signs suggesting the presence of elevated central venous pressure when cardiac causes are possible, suspected pericardial effusion, identification of tamponade physiology, and assessment of the size and function of the left ventricle when there is a suspicion of cardiomyopathy or cardiac failure.[6,7]

MODALITIES USED

Multiple modalities are used in combination to evaluate different areas and different functions of the heart. The 3 most important that are performed by emergency physicians are B-mode, M-mode, and Doppler. Bedside comprehensive echocardiography is requested occasionally to complement and address suspicions raised by goal-directed/emergency echocardiography. Additional information obtained may include quantitative analyses of valve function, detailed calculations of ejection fraction (EF), and tissue Doppler and diastolic function evaluations. More advanced modalities are beyond the scope of this article.

- *B-mode*. B-mode is also known as "brightness mode" or 2-dimensional (2D) ultrasound. Cardiac structures are shown in 2 dimensions and appear in shades of gray on the ultrasound monitor. It is ideal for real-time viewing of cardiac structures and their movements, and for the interpretation of cardiac function. Typically the real-time images are shown at a rate of 30 frames per second on the monitor. B-mode is the most common modality used in echocardiography, and is often used for the capture of still or video images.
- *M-mode*. This technology, also known as "motion mode," provides the opportunity to view and trace the motion and dimensions of heart structures with time. The M line, a very thin and linear area of ultrasound evaluation, allows faster image processing than the 30° sector used in 2D imaging, and can be precisely positioned through structures of interest. The rate of image capture with M-mode is 1800 frames per second (much faster than the human eye), which can discern variations in valve position, wall thickness, or chamber size over time. See **Figs. 1** and **2** for examples of M-mode tracings.
- *Applied Doppler technology*. "Doppler," as it is often described, actually includes several different subcategories including color Doppler, pulsed-wave Doppler, and continuous-wave Doppler. Each modality uses the same technology to measure heart parameters in a different way. The concept of Doppler is based on the ability of the ultrasound machine to measure the direction and magnitude of a frequency shift in cardiac muscle or blood flow relative to the transducer. This information is then translated into different colors or a graphic display of velocity magnitude on the ultrasound screen, depending on the subcategory being used. Color Doppler is most frequently used in emergency medicine to detect the presence of blood flow within a structure and to distinguish adjacent blood vessels (by showing different blood flow directions). Pulsed-wave and continuous-wave Doppler are used by emergency physicians with additional training, and their use is gradually increasing.

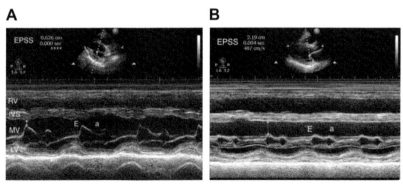

A   **B**

Fig. 1. E-point septal separation (EPSS). M-mode technology is used to trace the movement of the cardiac structures over time to more accurately estimate how closely the anterior leaflet of the mitral valve moves to the septum during left ventricular (LV) filling. The E wave (E) indicates the motion of the mitral valve toward the septum during LV filling. The A wave (a) indicates the motion of the mitral valve caused by atrial contraction. (*A*) An EPSS of 0.626 cm, indicating good systolic function. (*B*) The patient in this case. Her EPSS is calculated at 2.19 cm, indicating poor systolic function. IVS, interventricular septum; RV, right ventricle.

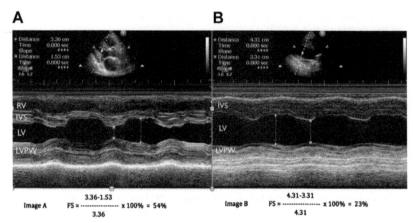

Fig. 2. Fractional shortening. M-mode evaluation of the LV chamber in parasternal long-axis (PSLA) view. (*A*) Evidence of wall thickening and endocardial excursion consistent with good systolic function. (*B*) The patient in this case. Both endocardial excursion and myocardial wall thickening are reduced, and fractional shortening is calculated at 23%. A normal value for fractional shortening is between 30% and 45%. IVS, interventricular septum; LV, left ventricle; LVPW, left ventricular posterior wall; RV, right ventricle.

WINDOWS USED

The main cardiac views obtained in transthoracic emergency echocardiography include the subcostal (subxiphoid), left parasternal (long and short axes), and apical windows. Subtle probe manipulations, such as angulation and rotation, can provide modified views of the heart chambers at different levels and perspectives. These different views may be used for identification of different wall segments, chambers, or valves, and may offer opportunities for Doppler interrogation and other physical or hemodynamic measurements. Each view may have technical challenges or feasibility issues in some patients. The indications and views listed in **Table 1** are discussed throughout this article.

TECHNICAL LIMITATIONS

Common technical challenges to acquiring adequate images in transthoracic echocardiography may include obesity, abdominal distension, a muscular chest wall, rapid breathing, air interference (chronic obstructive lung disease/hyperinflation/mechanical ventilation), small intercostal windows, chest wall tenderness, the presence of thoracic devices or ongoing thoracic procedures, subcutaneous emphysema, and pneumopericardium. Each window has its own diagnostic limitations and advantages. For example, the parasternal long-axis (PSLA) view is used to evaluate the thoracic aorta, but is limited to its very proximal section (the aortic root) and a small portion of the descending aorta as seen in cross section of the same view. Additional views may be used, such as the suprasternal view of the aortic arch or a modified apical 2-chamber view, depending on the skill of the operator and clinical information sought.

RETURN TO CASE 1

Your patient continues to be short of breath and tachypneic. Her blood pressure has decreased slightly, now at 79/44 mm Hg. Chest radiography is concerning for

Table 1
Summary of cardiac windows and important indications

Clinical Indication	Recommended Cardiac Window	Comments
Effusion detection	Subcostal PSLA	Often quickest and easiest to obtain Can differentiate pericardial from pleural effusion
RV evaluation	PSLA PSSA Apical 4-chamber	Evaluation for septal dyskinesis Look for "D sign" Comparison of chamber size
Global LV function[a]	PSLA	Ease of evaluation of mitral valve motion. Can also perform M-mode
Valve interrogation	Apical views	Allows for 0°–20° Doppler angle. Color or pulsed-wave modes
Volume assessment	Subcostal 4-chamber and IVC view (short or long)	Evaluation for respiratory variation of IVC and estimation of left ventricular end-diastolic area/volume
Shock/hypotension	Subcostal or PSLA	Use in combination with evaluation of aorta, pleura, and abdomen for free fluid to determine cause of shock
Proximal thoracic aortic disease	PSLA, modified apical 2, suprasternal view	Outflow >4 cm suggestive of proximal aortic disease (aneurysm) or intimal flap (dissection). Limited view of descending thoracic aorta. Suprasternal view may be used for evaluation of aortic arch *Note: TEE or CTA more sensitive and specific*
Cardiac arrest	Subcostal	Quick (<10 s) evaluation for presence of effusion, right ventricular strain, asystole

Abbreviations: CTA, computed tomographic angiography; IVC, inferior vena cava; LV, left ventricular; PSLA, parasternal long-axis view; PSSA, parasternal short-axis view; RV, right ventricular; TEE, transesophageal echocardiography.
[a] Detection of regional wall motion abnormalities requires multiple views.

pulmonary vascular congestion versus pneumonia. B-type natriuretic peptide is mildly elevated at 345 pg/mL. You suspect congestive heart failure, and turn to your bedside echocardiography skills for assistance.

Overall Cardiac Function

Overview
Cardiac function can be evaluated by multiple different modalities in the intensive care unit and the ED. Invasively obtained hemodynamic profiles are better suited to the intensive care setting, are time consuming, and are no more accurate than echocardiographic data.[8] Echocardiography is more convenient and provides a visual estimate of global cardiac function at the bedside. Features used in the visual estimation of left ventricular (LV) function are the change in chamber size, motion of endocardial surfaces or valves, and thickening of the myocardium. The normal left ventricle of the heart squeezes with a complex twisting mechanism, making precise measurements difficult. Geometric approximations and assumptions are made regarding the

shape and motion of the heart to assess ventricular function, which can contribute to variability in the final calculations of EF, stroke volume, and cardiac output. There are several ways to evaluate cardiac function with ultrasound, including quantitative and semiquantitative measurements, and visual estimates of systolic function. Other methods used in comprehensive echocardiography may include regional systolic wall motion grading, the use of tissue Doppler, and a more complex use of pulsed-wave Doppler to determine the Tei index of myocardial performance. The use of each method depends on the clinical scenario and skill of the sonographer. Multiple windows and modalities can be used to evaluate global systolic function, but in emergency echocardiography this may not be feasible.

Quantitative methods (ejection fraction)

LV systolic function is most frequently expressed as the EF. The EF is the percent volume change in ventricle size during systole, and is described by the equation EF = stroke volume/end-diastolic volume. Using a geometric model of a bullet shape, the endocardial surfaces of the left ventricle are traced from the base to the apex in both the apical 4-chamber view and the apical 2-chamber view to provide dimensions in 3 different planes. Diastolic volumetric measurements are subtracted from systolic measurements to determine the stroke volume. The stroke volume divided by the end-diastolic volume determines the EF. Many current ultrasound machines have packages available to assist with this calculation. For most clinical scenarios, though, an approximation is adequate and a formal calculation of EF is not necessary. In addition, it may be time consuming and beyond the scope of emergency medicine practice.

Semiquantitative methods

Other methods that closely approximate visual estimates of systolic function include fractional shortening (FS) and E-point septal separation (EPSS). Measurements of the changes in ventricular size are made in two planes (fractional area shortening) or in one plane (FS). The advantage of the semiquantitative approach is that measurements are easier to obtain than for EF while limiting the inherent human error or bias present with pure visual estimates.

- *EPSS.* An important marker of cardiac function is movement of the anterior leaflet of the mitral valve toward the interventricular septum during LV filling. In a heart with normal function, this leaflet should almost contact the interventricular septum. EPSS merely seeks to quantify how close the leaflet comes to the septum using M-mode evaluation of the mitral valve in the PSLA view. The E point is the top of the first waveform seen during diastole. The distance between the E point and the septum wall is called the EPSS. See **Fig. 1** for an example. Measurements greater than 0.6 to 1 cm for EPSS generally indicate severe systolic dysfunction (EF <30%). However, it should be noted that isolated or co-existing aortic insufficiency, dilated chambers, or mitral stenosis also increase the EPSS.[9,10] In one study, significant correlations between EPSS measurements and angiographic EF measurements were found except in cases with known mitral regurgitation and atrial fibrillation.[11]
- *Fractional shortening.* This method measures the fraction of a single LV diastolic dimension that is lost during systole. This fraction can be measured in various anatomic planes but with M-mode the parasternal views are most often used. Rather than using multiple different views and tracing the chambers as done with volumetric EF calculation, one simple view (typically the basal aspect of the LV diameter) and 2 measurements are all that are needed (see **Fig. 2**). The result of the comparison between systole and diastole dimensions is described

as a fraction or a percent change. A normal value for FS is approximately 30% to 45%. Fractional area shortening involves the loss in ventricular area (2 dimensions) between diastole and systole.

Visual estimates

Fortunately, the visual estimation of LV systolic function agrees with semiquantitative and quantitative measurements, allowing for accurate real-time assessments. Global systolic function assessments by emergency medicine physicians with focused training have good agreement with interpretations of the same echocardiography studies done by cardiologists.[12,13] Studies in adults and children have also shown good correlation between bedside estimation of LV function and semiquantitative measurements, with good interrater (blinded) agreement in visual LV function estimation when evaluation guidelines are followed.[11,14]

Visual estimates of systolic function are typically described as normal, moderately depressed, or poor. Emergency physicians tend to be relatively accurate at identifying normal or severely depressed cardiac function. However, the determination of moderately depressed cardiac function can be more difficult and there is a wider variation in this category. The 3 parameters that are most closely examined are mitral valve motion, myocardial wall thickening, and endocardial excursion. Each parameter is described here. The clinical interpretation depends on the clinical scenario, and a visual estimate of systolic function is often sufficient for the decision at hand. Patients may have comorbid cardiac conditions or acute cardiac dysfunction that may affect their response to therapeutic interventions such as acute volume loading.

- *Mitral valve motion.* The PSLA view is most often used for this indication. During diastolic filling, the anterior leaflet of the mitral valve moves upwards toward the interventricular septum. In a patient with normal LV function, the mitral valve should nearly contact the septum. On the other hand, patients with severely depressed LV function may have only a slight flicker of the mitral valve. Patients with moderately depressed function fall somewhere in between.
- *Myocardial wall thickening.* In a heart with normal cardiac function, the ventricular walls thicken significantly during systole and relax during diastole, as shown in Video 1. Patients with moderate and severely depressed dysfunction will show a decrease in this parameter. A visual gestalt is needed to estimate this parameter after viewing numerous echocardiograms of patients with varying degrees of cardiac function.
- *Endocardial excursion.* During systole the myocardium contracts, bringing the endocardial borders of the heart closer together as blood is ejected through the LV outflow tract. In a normal heart, the endocardial borders should come relatively close together, although no exact measurement is defined. A patient with moderately depressed or severely depressed cardiac function will have an echocardiogram that shows limited movement of the endocardial borders toward each other during systole. The ability to estimate this parameter is gained over time after viewing many echocardiograms of hearts with varying degrees of LV function.

A visual estimation scale of LV function that factored in the aforementioned parameters was shown to correlate well with bedside measurements of LV function and provided moderate interrater agreement.[11] See Videos 1–4 for examples.

One of the most valuable features of bedside global cardiac assessments is in ruling out severe systolic dysfunction. Cardiogenic shock carries a high morbidity and mortality, and early detection is crucial.[15] For example, the finding of severe systolic dysfunction in a patient with dyspnea and rales may be an indication for aggressive inotropic support. In another patient with hypotension of uncertain etiology, discovering normal to hyperdynamic systolic function may make it unlikely that the patient will require inotropic support or suffer from fluid toxicity in response to acute volume loading. Such a patient may instead tolerate and respond favorably to acute volume loading. Other causes of cardiogenic shock aside from severe systolic dysfunction include tamponade, severe valvular dysfunction, and ventricular septal wall rupture.

Case 1 Conclusion

A bedside echocardiogram shows evidence of severely depressed cardiac function by visual gestalt and an EPSS is calculated at 1.4 cm. The patient is admitted for diuresis and improves symptomatically. A comprehensive echocardiogram obtained the next day shows an EF of 15% to 20%.

Special Circumstances

While emergency physicians can accurately discriminate between depressed and normal LV systolic function by visual estimation, there are several additional circumstances that should be noted.

- *Cardiomyopathies.* During evaluation for systolic function, evidence of cardiomyopathies can often be found. The two most common are shown here. Dilated cardiomyopathy appears as thin-walled, dilated chambers with poor systolic function. Hypertrophic cardiomyopathy appears as thick ventricle walls (>15 mm) with impaired relaxation (diastolic dysfunction), and usually intact systolic function unless it is at the end stage. A detailed discussion of the cardiomyopathies is beyond the scope of this article, but is mentioned in the event it is seen, so that the sonographer can become familiar with their appearance and arrange appropriate subspecialty consultation and follow-up if found. See **Fig. 3**, and Videos 5 and 6 for examples of dilated and hypertrophic cardiomyopathy.
- *Diastolic dysfunction.* it is important to remember that diastolic function is usually evaluated by comprehensive echocardiography, and a detailed discussion is beyond the scope of this article. Diastolic dysfunction can be evaluated at the bedside using M-mode of the mitral valve leaflet movement or Doppler

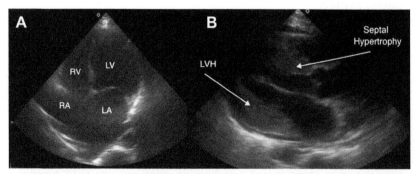

Fig. 3. Cardiomyopathies. Compare and contrast the thin-walled, dilated chambers of a patient with dilated cardiomyopathy (*A*; apical 4-chamber view) with the thick-walled chambers of the patient with hypertrophic cardiomyopathy (*B*; PSLA view). See Videos 5 and 6. LA, left atrium; LV, left ventricle; LVH, left ventricular hypertrophy; RA, right atrium; RV, right ventricle.

interrogation of valvular flow. Normal filling of the left ventricle (diastole) begins with, and is predominantly achieved by, isovolemic relaxation of the left ventricle. The rest of the LV filling is supplemented by atrial contraction. The anterior leaflet opening (using M-mode) or blood flow velocity (using pulsed-wave Doppler) during isovolemic relaxation phase of diastole is depicted as the E wave. The second and smaller A wave represents movement/blood flow due to the left atrial contraction phase of diastole. A reduction or reversal of the normal E/A wave ratio indicates impaired relaxation of the left ventricle. It should be noted that up to a third of cases of heart failure is caused by diastolic dysfunction, and that a visual estimation of normal systolic function does not rule out the possible presence of diastolic dysfunction or heart failure. See **Fig. 4** and Video 7 for an example of pulsed-wave Doppler imaging in a patient with diastolic dysfunction.

- *Hyperdynamic heart*. Hyperdynamic heart refers to the near obliteration of the ventricular cavity during systole, and may represent an elevated EF but not necessarily an increased stroke volume. This condition does not necessarily refer to the rate of contractions but rather to its vigor. Hyperdynamic heart activity can be found in hyperthyroidism or adrenergic surge states (after epinephrine/dopamine administration or certain drug overdoses). It may also be a compensatory response to poor oxygen-carrying abilities such as in low-volume states or anemia. A hyperdynamic heart effectively rules out systolic dysfunction as the cause of a patient's symptoms. A well-filled hyperdynamic heart can be found in distributive shock states such as sepsis or anaphylaxis. A barely filled hyperdynamic heart suggests hypovolemia or hemorrhage, and a search for hemorrhage or vascular emergency should be pursued based on the clinical context. See Video 7 for an example of a hyperdynamic heart in the PSLA view.

CASE 2

Your next patient has persistent hiccups for 4 days. He has a history of chronic renal failure and has received all of his hemodialysis treatments as scheduled this week. He endorses generalized fatigue but denies chest pain, vomiting, or abnormal colored

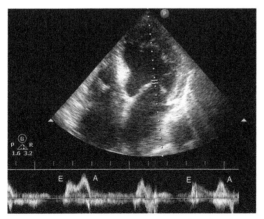

Fig. 4. Diastolic dysfunction. A pulsed-wave Doppler apical 4-chamber view in a patient with impaired cardiac relaxation and evidence of diastolic dysfunction. Note the reversal of the E/A wave ratio, indicating that there is a greater contribution to LV filling from atrial contraction due to the increased resistance to passive flow into the LV during diastole. Refer also to **Fig. 13** for diastolic dysfunction.

stool. On examination, he has stable vital signs and an unremarkable cardiovascular examination with the exception of mild jugular venous distension. He has clear lungs bilaterally and a nontender abdomen. You order a chest radiograph and note mild pulmonary vascular congestion, no peridiaphragmatic lesions, and cardiomegaly that is unchanged compared with his previous chest radiographs. His electrocardiogram (ECG) shows low-voltage QRS complexes but no PR or ST segment abnormalities. Due to suspicion of pericardial effusion, you proceed with bedside cardiac ultrasound and it confirms the diagnosis. Next, you carefully look at his heart chambers.

Pericardial Effusion Detection

Overview

The normal pericardial space usually contains a small volume (5–10 mL) of pericardial fluid, which functions as a lubricant between the visceral and parietal pericardium. The pericardial space of the normal adult heart can hold up to 50 mL of pericardial fluid before clinically significant elevations in intrapericardial pressure occur. Small accumulations may be barely discernible without the use of multiple windows.

- *Clinical clues.* The spectrum of symptoms and signs is variable and can include dyspnea, chest pain, and/or tachycardia. However, there are other vague symptoms such as nausea and singultus that may indicate the presence of an underlying effusion. The emergency physician must therefore be vigilant about comorbid conditions that are typically associated with pericardial effusion accumulations. A high index of suspicion will lower the threshold for the evaluation and detection of pericardial effusion.
- *Sonographic appearance.* Pericardial effusions are usually echolucent (black) and contrast sharply with the echogenicity of fibrous pericardium and myocardium. Some pericardial accumulations are more challenging to discern, as they may have a heterogeneous gray appearance if composed of clotting blood or other debris. Benign epicardial fat is usually located anteriorly, and can be mistaken for a small pericardial effusion.
- *Sonographic views.* In a trauma setting, the subxiphoid view is commonly used and is often the easiest view to obtain. However, the PSLA view offers the advantage in more accurately differentiating pericardial effusion from pleural effusion, and can help to further evaluate the size of the effusion and its hemodynamic effects. The apical 4-chamber view may be used as well, especially when considering ultrasound-guided pericardiocentesis. See **Figs. 5** and **6**, and Videos 8 and 9 for parasternal views of a moderate-sized pericardial effusion.
- *Size.* A pericardial effusion is usually quantified as small, moderate, or large. Effusion volume size can be estimated as being small if the distance between the epicardium to pericardium is less than 0.5 cm; moderate if 0.5 to 2 cm, and large if greater than 2 cm. By obtaining multiple views of the heart, one can increase confidence in ruling out a small or loculated effusion. Small effusions are usually confined to the posterior space. However, moderate to large effusions tend to envelope the heart and have a greater width. These effusions may be confirmed using a single cardiac window. Larger effusions increase the likelihood of acute tamponade physiology and need for emergent pericardial drainage. **Fig. 7**A and Video 10 show pericardial effusions of 3 different sizes from a subxiphoid view.

Etiology

There are multiple causes of pericardial fluid accumulations, which can roughly be divided into traumatic and nontraumatic mechanisms.

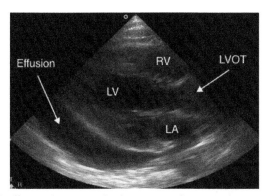

Fig. 5. Pericardial effusion (PSLA view), showing moderate to large pericardial effusion without evidence of cardiac tamponade. This particular patient had a history of end-stage renal disease. Despite the large size, no significant hemodynamic effects are seen, due to its chronicity. See Video 8. LA, left atrium; LV, left ventricle; LVOT, left ventricular outflow tract; RV, right ventricle.

- *Trauma.* Cardiac ultrasound is part of the Focused Assessment with Sonography in Trauma (FAST). Examination of cardiac windows is especially important in cases of penetrating injuries near the heart or in truncal injuries where the trajectory of a bullet is uncertain. With blunt trauma, in addition to pericardial effusion detection, it is also advised to examine for decreased cardiac activity caused by myocardial contusion.[1] In cases of blunt trauma where the presence of a pericardial effusion may be an incidental but preexisting finding, an expeditious query of previous records or comparison of previous imaging may be required. In these cases, a pericardial effusion is considered a false positive if it is erroneously considered a consequence of acute traumatic injury. Conversely, penetrating injuries to the pericardium and heart can lead to spillage of blood and negligible pericardial accumulations. In such a case, the nonvisualization of pericardial fluid during FAST should be reported as such and not be considered a definitive

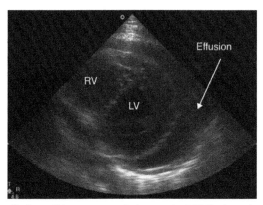

Fig. 6. Pericardial effusion. This parasternal short-axis (PSSA) view shows a moderate to large pericardial effusion. Note that there is no evidence of right ventricular collapse or developing cardiac tamponade. See Video 9. LV, left ventricle; RV, right ventricle.

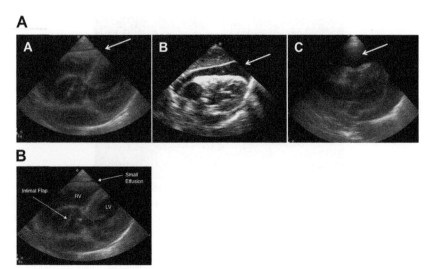

Fig. 7. (*A*) Pericardial effusion size comparison (*arrows*). (*A*) A small anterior pericardial effusion. (*B*) An example of a moderate-sized effusion. (*C*) Presence of a large effusion. All views are subcostal. Note that a small anterior pericardial effusion is sometimes confused with an epicardial fat pad. (*B*) Aortic dissection with small anterior effusion. This subcostal view is an enlargement of image *A* in the previous figure. It shows a small anterior effusion from an ascending aortic dissection. The intimal flap of the dissection is seen here as well. Although the effusion is small, the mechanism suggests potential for rapid accumulation and development of cardiac tamponade. See Video 10.

"ruling out" of cardiac injury. In the penetrating trauma setting, smaller fluid collections are more likely to provoke tamponade physiology and hemodynamic instability. A hypovolemic patient will have lower right heart pressures and, thus, cardiac tamponade physicology can occur with much lower pericardial pressures resulting from smaller effusions.

- *Nontrauma.* Many possible causes are appropriate to consider in the absence of trauma and may include inflammatory, infectious, malignant, or autoimmune conditions as well as aortic dissection. Pericardial effusions are also commonly seen in patients with renal failure, lupus, cancer, acquired immunodeficiency syndrome, and pregnancy. Transudative effusions tend to appear similar to traumatic effusions (echolucent or black), whereas exudative or malignant effusions can vary widely in their appearance.

Tamponade physiology

The presence of a pericardial fluid accumulation is considered a necessary but not sufficient condition for the clinical diagnosis of tamponade. For a critically ill patient with a pericardial effusion, it is essential to be aware of the clinical factors affecting the development of cardiac tamponade.

- *Identification.* Tamponade physiology is most commonly identified by decreased right ventricular (RV) size with early diastolic collapse and late expansion (specific not sensitive), as seen in **Fig. 8**A and B, and Videos 11 and 12. This condition is a result of an elevation in intrapericardial pressure limiting RV free wall expansion and thus compromising LV filling and cardiac output. Other features suggestive of tamponade physiology include right atrial collapse at early diastole, as seen in **Fig. 9** and Video 13 (most sensitive feature). This finding becomes more specific

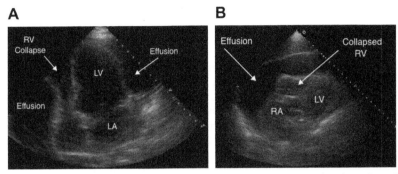

Fig. 8. (*A*) Apical 4-chamber pericardial tamponade. This apical 4-chamber view shows a moderate-sized pericardial effusion with collapse of the right ventricle (RV), indicating high intrapericardial pressures and subsequent cardiac tamponade. See Video 11. (*B*) Subcostal view of pericardial tamponade. A large pericardial effusion is seen with compression of all heart chambers, including the RV. See Video 12. LA, left atrium; LV, left ventricle; RA, right atrium.

when right atrial diastolic collapse persists.[16] Of note, right atrial collapse may also be found in the presence of a pleural effusion or hypovolemia. Finally, tamponade physiology should be suspected when there is also minimal to absent respiratory diameter variation of the inferior vena cava (IVC). Technical limitations to tamponade detection include the presence of tachycardia, tachypnea, or challenging windows due to body habitus, making it difficult to confidently distinguish diastolic and systolic phases. If the sonographer is uncertain, M-mode technology may be used to evaluate for subtle posterior movement of the RV free wall during diastole in the PSLA view.

- *Rate of accumulation.* The pericardium is mostly fibrous and has a limited degree of elasticity. Gradual increases in pericardial fluid volume and intrapericardial

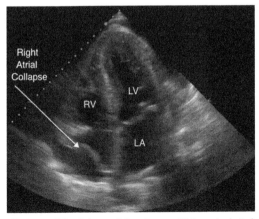

Fig. 9. Pericardial effusion with right atrial collapse. This apical 4-chamber view shows a moderate-sized effusion with evidence of increasing intrapericardial pressures causing collapse of the right atrium. The right ventricle (RV) size is normal because the right ventricular diastolic pressure is greater than the intrapericardial pressure. See Video 13. LA, left atrium; LV, left ventricle.

pressure can be tolerated until the relatively low pressure of the thin right heart walls is exceeded. A pericardial effusion can accumulate insidiously or suddenly, depending on the clinical context. As a general rule, rapidly accumulating effusions tend to have more notable physiologic effects. For example, the chronic effusion of a patient with renal failure may not affect hemodynamic parameters until it is quite large. By contrast, a small traumatic pericardial bloody effusion may quickly lead to hemodynamic collapse in an otherwise healthy patient, due to its rapid rate of accumulation.

- *Clinical decision making*. In the unstable patient (eg, cardiac arrest, chest pain, or shock), when a significant pericardial effusion is detected then clinical tamponade should be considered the likely cause of the patient's instability. If tamponade physiology is still uncertain or suspected and the patient is quasi-stable, emergency comprehensive echocardiography and cardiology consultation are suggested. Comprehensive studies usually perform contemporaneous electrocardiographic monitoring to definitively determine systolic and diastolic phases. Another sign of developing tamponade is paradoxic septal wall motion. Detection of tamponade may also require the use of Doppler interrogation to detect increased triscuspid flow velocity or decreased mitral forward flow velocity with inspiration. Emergent pericardiocentesis (nontrauma setting) or pericardial window placement (preferred) is the definitive treatment of tamponade.

Pericardiocentesis

If pericardiocentesis is indicated in the ED, real-time ultrasound guidance is suggested to improve success and reduce complication rates.[17,18] Direct needle guidance and entry into the pericardial space, a reduction of pericardial fluid volume, and improved right chamber expansion can be seen sonographically. The most common methods are a direct in-line approach with the subxiphoid view or an apical approach with sonographic evaluation of the subxiphoid view simultaneously.

Case 2 Conclusion

This patient is found to have a moderate-sized pericardial effusion without evidence of tamponade physiology. His blood pressure remains stable and the patient is admitted for further workup of the source of his effusion. Consideration is also made for placement of a pigtail catheter for drainage of the effusion.

Pitfalls

There are several tips to remember when evaluating a patient for a pericardial effusion or signs of tamponade.

- *Chronic pulmonary hypertension*. It must be noted that in conditions causing chronically elevated right-sided chamber pressure, there may not be right atrial or RV collapse until the intrapericardial pressure is very high. Such conditions may show a pericardial effusion with a distended right atrium and ventricle, RV hypertrophy, and plethora of the IVC. Consider the patient's previous history when making this determination.
- Right-sided heart chamber pressures are more easily exceeded (leading to collapse) in conditions of volume depletion.
- *Differentiation from pleural effusion*. To the untrained eye, a left pleural effusion can be mistaken for a pericardial effusion. The pericardial space surrounds most of the heart except at the base and stops near the atrioventricular sulcus and anterior to the adjacent descending aorta. Unloculated fluid in the pericardial

space is contained within the pericardial space, and does not appear posterior to the descending aorta or atrioventricular sulcus on the parasternal view (as seen in **Fig. 10** and Video 14). Fluid seen posterior to the descending aorta is considered pleural fluid in the left thorax. Pleural fluid can therefore be confused with a pericardial fluid (false positive) if the descending aorta is not used as a reference point.

CASE 3

A 56-year-old man experiences sudden pleuritic chest pain and shortness of breath. He is mildly hypoxic at 92% but his chest radiograph shows clear lungs and no cardiomegaly. His ECG shows tachycardia but no classic signs of ischemia or infarction. Emergency echocardiogram shows no pericardial effusion, normal LV systolic function, and something else...

Right Ventricular Size and Function

Anatomy

The right ventricle of the normal adult heart has a basal width that is less than 60% that of the left ventricle. The normal left ventricle is more muscular and its apex is bluntly curved, occupying two-thirds of the heart's apex. By contrast, the right ventricle's apex tapers sharply when viewed with the apical 4-window. The RV free wall is thin and creates a relatively low-pressure chamber. The interventricular septal wall is therefore contoured (bowed) toward the right ventricle. The normal right ventricle has a crescentic (semilunar) appearance on the parasternal short-axis (PSSA) view and is significantly smaller than the left ventricle.

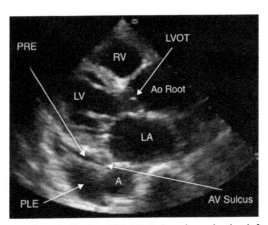

Fig. 10. Pericardial and pleural effusion. This PSLA view shows both a left pleural and a pericardial effusion. The descending aorta (A) is a key anatomic landmark. The pericardium attaches to the heart at the atrioventricular (AV) sulcus, limiting the expansion of the pericardial effusion (PRE) and thus helps to differentiate it from a pleural effusion (PLE), which is also seen here. Pericardial fluid accumulations do not extend posterior to the descending aorta (A). A left pleural effusion extends behind the descending aorta and thus is distinguished from the pericardial effusion. Note also that the aortic (Ao) root is dilated (>4 cm), which is suggestive of an ascending thoracic aortic aneurysm. The left atrium (LA) is enlarged as well. See Video 14. LV, left ventricle; LVOT, left ventricular outflow tract; RV, right ventricle.

Echocardiographic signs

- *RV dilation.* As previously mentioned, the right ventricle is typically smaller (<60%) than the left ventricle under normal conditions. However, with increases in right-sided pressure or volume, the right ventricle may enlarge to equal or exceed the size of the left ventricle. The causes of RV dilation (acute cor pulmonale) are multiple and may include pulmonary embolus (PE), primary pulmonary hypertension, chronic obstructive pulmonary obstruction, elevated intrathoracic pressure from mechanical ventilation, RV infarction, certain cardiomyopathies, and other conditions. See **Fig. 11, Fig. 12**A and B, and Videos 15–20 for examples of RV dilation.
- *Paradoxic septal motion.* In a normal heart, the higher pressures of the left ventricle move the septal wall bowed toward the right ventricle throughout a normal cardiac cycle. With RV strain, RV enlargement due to volume or pressure increases can compete with or may even exceed the LV pressures. Significant RV pressure may straighten the septal wall or even cause it to bow toward the left ventricle, as seen in **Fig. 13**, an M-mode tracing in the PSLA view. This abnormal septal motion is also called septal dyskinesis. The resulting decrease in LV filling may lead to significant reductions in cardiac output.[19]
- *Decreased IVC respiratory variation.* Elevated right-sided pressure or volume will reduce the variability of the IVC during a normal respiratory cycle and give the appearance of physiologic fluid overload; this is discussed in more detail in a later section. However, it should be noted that the presence of decreased respiratory variation as a result of pulmonary hypertension should not be automatically interpreted as fluid overload. Fluid administration may still be an important intervention in certain cases, including acute PE.
- *Other findings.* One study determined 100% hospital mortality for pulmonary embolism when shock signs were accompanied by echocardiographic findings of diastolic LV impairment (E/A wave <1), RV hypokinesis, RV/LV ratio >1, and end-diastolic RV diameter >3 cm.[20] Another study determined that in normotensive patients with PE and RV systolic overload, tricuspid velocity and troponin level were better at risk-stratifying patients than RV to LV diameter ratio.[21] The bottom line is that for patients in extremis with acute RV enlargement signs, massive pulmonary embolism should be considered. When the patient is not in

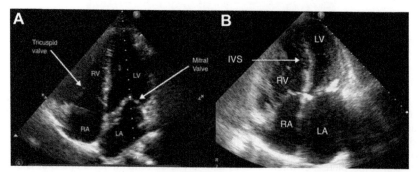

Fig. 11. Right ventricular strain (4-chamber). (*A*) A normal apical 4-chamber view. (*B*) Apical 4-chamber view of a patient with elevated right heart pressures. Notice the enlargement of the right ventricle (RV) and bowing of the septum toward the left ventricle (LV) in (*B*). See Videos 15 and 16. LA, left atrium; IVS, interventricular septum; RA, right atrium.

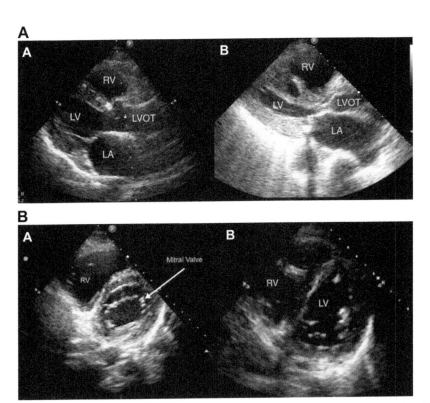

Fig. 12. (*A*) Right ventricular strain (PSLA). (*A*) A normal PSLA view. (*B*) A dilated right ventricle (RV) compressing the left ventricle (LV), due to high right-sided pressures. A dilated left atrium (LA) is also seen. Notice how the interventricular septum has shifted toward the LV, compromising filling. See Videos 17 and 18. LVOT, left ventricular outflow tract. (*B*) Right ventricular strain (PSSA). (*A*) A normal PSSA view, showing a circular left ventricle (LV) at the level of the mitral valve. (*B*) A dilated right ventricle (RV) causing shift of the septal wall, and a D-shaped LV caused by the elevated right heart pressure. See Videos 19 and 20.

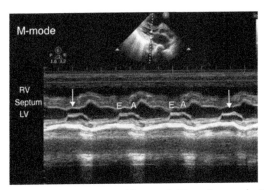

Fig. 13. RV strain (M-mode). This parasternal long-axis M-mode snapshot shows evidence of elevated right heart pressure and septal dyskinesis. The E and A waves represent the diastolic phases of passive LV filling and atrial contraction, respectively. In this case, the E and A wave are of similar size, consistent with diastolic dysfunction. Note that in diastole the septum shifts toward the LV (*arrows*), due to the abnormally elevated right heart pressures, as indicated by the arrows.

extremis, more advanced emergency echocardiography parameters and biomarkers can be used for risk stratification of suspected or diagnosed pulmonary embolism.

- *Acute versus chronic.* Right ventricular hypertrophy, defined as an RV free wall thickness greater than 5 mm, usually suggests chronic RV pressure elevation. This condition occurs because chronic RV pressure increases lead to RV enlargement with RV hypertrophy, and may include right atrial dilation as well. By contrast, an acute increase in RV wall tension may compromise perfusion, leading to ischemia-related reductions in RV systolic function without an increase in RV free wall thickness. See **Fig. 14** and Video 21 for an example.

Diagnostic utility

- *PE.* Emergency transthoracic echocardiography rarely makes a definitive diagnosis of massive pulmonary embolism or a thrombus in transit.[22,23] Unlike transesophageal echocardiography, which can detect thrombi in the central pulmonary arterial tree, transthoracic echocardiography merely searches for signs of pressure buildup from a massive or submassive pulmonary embolism lodged in the proximal or lobar pulmonary arteries.[24] A large PE is needed to achieve this effect, and occlusion of more than 30% of the pulmonary arterial tree usually can lead to RV dilation and evidence of poor RV function.[25]
- *Echocardiography.* Echocardiography should not be used to reduce the suspicion or stop the search for a clinically significant PE, as it is not considered a good screening test for this diagnosis.[26] However, echocardiography combined with venous ultrasound showed improved sensitivity when severe dyspnea or high pretest suspicion existed.[27] Computed tomographic angiography (CTA) of the thorax is still the preferred imaging study to definitively make or exclude the diagnosis of pulmonary embolism.
- *Undifferentiated shock and hypotension.* In patients with undifferentiated shock and hypotension, emergency echocardiography searches for previously

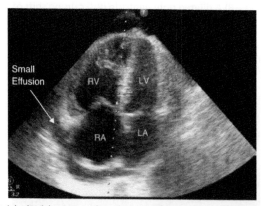

Fig. 14. Right ventricle (RV) hypertrophy. This apical 4-chamber view shows prominent dilation of the right atrium (RA) and RV compared with the left heart chambers. The enlarged RV now occupies most of the cardiac apex. The RV free wall is thickened, suggesting chronic pulmonary hypertension. A small pericardial effusion is seen lateral to the RA and RV. Given the chronically elevated right heart pressures, tamponade is less likely to occur, as it will require higher intrapericardial pressures to collapse this RV. See Video 21. LA, left atrium; LV, left ventricle.

discussed pericardial effusion, global heart function, and then for RV enlarge-ment. If RV dilation is discovered, the next step is to determine whether it is acute or chronic. Chronic RV dysfunction and enlargement are suggested if there is associated left-sided dilation or dysfunction, RV hypertrophy, or right atrial dila-tion. Both RV pressure and volume overload conditions can lead to enlargement of the right ventricle with straightening or bowing of the interventricular septum into the left ventricle. In the cardiac arrest scenario, a massive PE is definitely a possibility, and emergency echocardiography screening may be the only diag-nostic imaging option available.[28] RV strain can explain associated IVC plethora, and this makes volume assessment by using echocardiography challenging. The findings of RV dilation and ischemia-induced RV dysfunction are important risk-stratification criteria in patients with confirmed acute submassive PE. Its pres-ence portends increased short-term mortality and long-term morbidity.[26,29-34] Primary RV infarction also may show up as RV hypokinesis, but is commonly associated with LV inferior wall segment motion abnormalities.

- RV dysfunction can be found in as many as 40% of hemodynamically stable cases of confirmed PE. Other studies report up to 20% of confirmed PE cases have normal echocardiographic findings. Overall the finding of RV enlargement in an unstable patient should strongly place submassive PE on the differential diagnosis and consideration for definitive diagnosis.[21,35]

Case 3 Conclusion

The patient is found to have evidence of RV dilation on both the apical 4-chamber and PSSA views during evaluation by bedside echo. CTA of the chest is obtained, identi-fying a PE in the right pulmonary artery. The patient continues to decompensate with declining respiratory status and worsening hypotension. Thrombolytic agents are given based on the patient's computed tomography findings and evidence of RV strain. The patient is transferred to the medical intensive care unit for further care.

CASE 4

A 47-year-old man collapses in the airport while transferring flights. The prehospital team appropriately initiates Advanced Cardiopulmonary Life Support (ACLS) protocol and after 10 minutes he arrives in your ED undergoing active cardiopulmonary resus-citation (CPR) by medics. He is morbidly obese. You notice an atrioventricular fistula and his left arm as well as some bilateral lower extremity edema. Pulses are very diffi-cult to palpate because of the patient's body habitus, and a manual blood pressure is unobtainable. The new attending to your staff wants to use the ultrasound machine to look at his heart quickly.

Cardiac Arrest

Overview

Bedside cardiac ultrasound can be used to determine the presence and degree of cardiac activity in situations whereby identification of a palpable pulse is uncertain. Though not explicitly stated in ACLS guidelines, emergency physicians have realized that the usefulness of goal-directed emergency echocardiography is exemplified in the pulseless electrical activity (PEA) and asystole cardiac arrest situation. During pulse checks, a brief viewing of the heart can identify cardiac activity, screen for peri-cardial effusions and tamponade, look for significant right heart strain, or evaluate for severe volume depletion. The cardiac ultrasound views must be promptly started and skillfully obtained during the 5-second "pulse check." It should supplement and not interrupt the course of the resuscitation. The subcostal view is typically easiest to obtain during insufflation in a mechanically ventilated patient. Serial heart evaluations can be performed during the course of the resuscitation.[36–40] See Video 22 for an example of a subcostal view to evaluate for the presence of cardiac function.

Advantages

- *Lack of interruptions with CPR.* There is minimal interruption on resuscitative efforts in exchange for the critical and time-sensitive information that is provided to the treating physicians. A quick look of several seconds on the subxiphoid cardiac window may give more information than attempting to palpate a pulse in a patient with a difficult body habitus.[39] Serial evaluations will show the return of spontaneous circulation, or if the heart activity deteriorates or is refractory to resuscitative efforts.
- *Identification of life-threatening pathology.* Recent ACLS guidelines list several potentially reversible causes that must be considered in the patient presenting in PEA.[41,42] Emergency echocardiography can quickly identify several of the causes of severe shock, including pericardial effusion/tamponade, evidence of RV strain (PE), and signs of cardiac underfilling or severe hypovolemia. The time-sensitive ruling-in and ruling-out of severe cardiac conditions can guide therapeutic interventions, improve resuscitation efforts, and may provide more informed decision making on each critically ill patient.[3,43–45]
- *Improvement in resuscitative efforts.* Once cardiac activity is identified, echo can be used to guide resuscitative efforts. Serial examinations can identify progression in hemodynamic status or contractility following the initiation of intravenous fluid resuscitation or adrenergic agents.[46]
- *Patient safety.* The days of the blind pericardiocentesis attempts during an undifferentiated PEA resuscitation are long gone. Furthermore, ultrasound can be used to guide the procedure if one is detected. It may also assist in determining the presence of transcutaneous or transvenous pacer capture in the right clinical scenario.

Survival

When cardiac ultrasound shows no ventricular activity and there is asystole on the cardiac monitor after full ACLS resuscitative attempts by paramedics, survival is rare.[39,47,48] Other signs of failure of resuscitation include the development of coagulating blood and isolated atrial and valve movement without organized ventricular activity.[40] These small, isolated valve movements are not the same as organized cardiac contractions, and the resuscitation should not be continued based on these findings alone. It must also be noted that reversible and transient myocardial stunning is a phenomenon that exists and may result from acute coronary hypoperfusion, noncardiac causes such as intracranial hemorrhage, acute drug toxicity, and others.[49–51] Finding persistent asystole during serial ultrasound evaluations (while full resuscitative efforts continue) helps to better rule out periarrest transient myocardial stunning and confirms an unsuccessful resuscitation.[52,53]

Pediatric considerations

The primary reasons for pediatric arrests are usually not cardiac but are due to respiratory complications and insufficiency.[54] The detection of pulses during pulse checks can be very challenging in the pediatric periarrest time. Emergency echocardiography evaluates pump function as part of the circulation assessment.[55]

Case 4 Conclusion

Subcostal cardiac views are obtained rapidly during pulse checks, and indicate that despite the absence of definite palpable pulses, the patient does have evidence of cardiac activity on your bedside echo. A stat basic metabolic panel is ordered and shows the presence of hyperkalemia at 7.3 mEq/L. The patient is treated with calcium, bicarbonate, insulin, and glucose, with improvement of his hemodynamic status. Nephrology is consulted for emergent dialysis. The patient is discharged 5 days later with no evidence of neurologic dysfunction.

CASE 5

A 45-year-old man with cardiac disease and diabetes mellitus presents with weakness, hypotension, and tachycardia. He appears emaciated. His serum glucose, anion gap, and acetone levels are all elevated. Bedside echocardiography is notable for a hyperdynamic left ventricle and an IVC diameter of 2 cm with minimal respiratory size variation. Based on the patient's history and echocardiographic findings, what is his volume status?

Volume Assessment

Overview

The volume status of patients presenting to the ED with critical illness or injury is often unclear. Traditionally, physicians have relied on their physical examination findings to help make this determination. However, physical signs are not always accurate in the detection of hypovolemia.[56,57] Other traditional methods have proved unreliable as well. A recent meta-analysis has shown that invasively obtained hemodynamic information such as central venous pressure (CVP) has a poor correlation with actual volume status.[50] The potential consequences of inaccurate judgment of volume status are not minor. Acute volume loading can provoke fluid overload in patients with an unsuspected primary cardiogenic etiology. Suboptimal volume resuscitation can prolong end-organ hypoperfusion, dysfunction, or failure. Bedside cardiac ultrasound aims to noninvasively evaluate pump filling as well as filling of the IVC, the main conduit of venous blood return to the heart.

Physiology

There has been much research on the use of the IVC in estimating intravascular volume. The IVC is a distensible and collapsible vein returning venous blood to the right atrium of the heart. The two most often described sonographic parameters in determining volume status are IVC size and respiratory variation. Both features are influenced by pressure and volume changes within the heart. These changes may be related to myocardial compliance, valve function, intrathoracic pressure, pericardial pressure, or intra-abdominal pressure, and all are factors that influence IVC respiratory dynamics.

- Pump filling. Pump filling represents LV preload, and can be appreciated and quantified as LV end-diastolic area or LV end-diastolic volume. It can also be visually estimated during emergency echocardiography. Hypervolemia is often associated with increased LV end-diastolic dimensions (dilated left ventricle) and depressed systolic function. One cardiac ultrasound feature that is highly suggestive of hypovolemia includes PSSA views showing touching ("kissing") papillary muscles during systole. Another feature is very low to absent end-diastolic LV volumes when using the parasternal long, subcostal or apical 4-chamber views. Classic severe hypovolemia signs can also include near to complete emptying of the heart, hypercontractility, and rapid contractions. Keep in mind that some patients may have preexisting systolic dysfunction or may be unable to mount a compensatory rate increase in response to low LV preload if on certain medications, including β-blockers.

- *IVC size.* In previous studies, several attempts were made to correlate CVP with IVC diameter and respiratory variation. However, these IVC size measurements alone as an indicator of fluid status have fallen out of favor, due to their unreliability. One of the first studies to support this finding showed a significant overlap in IVC diameter between normal subjects and those with cardiac disease, indicating that size alone is not a reliable indicator of fluid status.[58] The same study also found that patients with isolated right heart disease had distinctly lower respiratory variations in IVC diameter when compared with their healthy counterparts.[58] Therefore, variation in IVC size was thought to hold some promise as an estimation of right-sided filling pressures. Note that right-sided filling pressures are affected by several factors, including pulmonary hypertension, myocardial compliance, valve function, presence of pericardial effusion and/or PE, and general hydration status of the patient. Each assessment must be taken within the clinical context of the patient, and assumptions should not be made about the hydration status based on isolated IVC measurements. See **Fig. 15**, and Videos 23 and 24 for a comparison between a plethoric and collapsible IVC.

- *IVC respiratory variation.* Usually there is some degree of variation in IVC diameter during each breathing cycle. However, the nature of the variation differs depending on the mode of ventilation. During spontaneous breathing, inhalation decreases intrathoracic pressure, causing the return of venous blood to the right atrium and a brief decrease in IVC diameter; this is also called IVC collapsibility. On the other hand, patients being mechanically ventilated show the opposite effects. Positive pressure ventilation increases intrathoracic pressure, causing less inflow of blood to the lungs, thus increasing the IVC diameter; this is also known as IVC distensibility. Some studies use IVC distensibility in monitoring acute volume-loading adjustments in mechanically ventilated patients.[59,60] The absolute value of the change of IVC size is more important than the direction of change. Usually with volume depletion, the change in size of the IVC is more dramatic than in normovolemic or hypervolemic states.

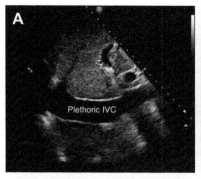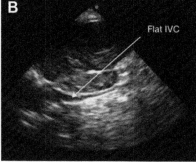

Fig. 15. Inferior vena cava (IVC) evaluation. (*A*) A subcostal longitudinal view of a dilated, plethoric IVC. By contrast, (*B*) shows an IVC that is nearly fully collapsed. This appearance often indicates hypovolemia, but clinical correlation is needed, as discussed in the text. See Videos 23 and 24.

The measurement of IVC collapsibility is referred to as the caval index, often expressed as a percentage. The caval index is calculated by the equation:

$$Caval\ Index = \left(IVC_{exp} - IVC_{insp}\right)/IVC_{exp} \times 100\%$$

A high caval index in general indicates a higher probability of hypovolemia, although the cutoff values vary depending on which study is cited. Several other studies have shown good interrater agreement in the calculated caval index measurements when compared with visual estimates of the same parameters.[11,12,61] **Fig. 16** shows a comparison between a high and low caval indices by M-mode evaluation.

Clinical utility
In a study of acute volume loading of hypotensive ED patients without signs of congestive heart failure, no fluid toxicity was provoked even in patients with low caval index before volume load. IVC diameters increased with volume loading as well. Baseline high caval indices acutely decreased (filled up) whereas low caval indices at baseline remained low.[11] When IVC plethora is encountered, a search for signs of right and left heart strain or effusion with tamponade is strongly suggested. IVC size and caval index are influenced by pressure elevation and may not be due to a state of volume overload unless other clinical signs (eg, pulmonary vascular congestion) are present. When there is an elevated caval index (increased IVC collapsibility), low pressures and low volume states are more likely.

Limitations of sonographic evaluation of the IVC for determination of fluid status

- *Correlation with CVP unreliable.* Previous studies have attempted to show correlations of IVC size and dynamics with central venous pressure measurements.[58,62–64] Acute fluid loading and fluid removal studies have demonstrated temporally associated acute changes in IVC size and dynamics, but these have been performed in a myriad of subjects (healthy, mechanically ventilated, cardiac diseases, sepsis, and right heart strain).[59,60,65,66] It must be emphasized that in clinical studies IVC dynamics and size have been mainly correlated with right heart pressure measurements rather than volume states.[58,67,68] A recent study by Brennan and colleagues[69] reassessed the previously used model that categorized CVP into 5-mm Hg ranges based on IVC findings, and found it to

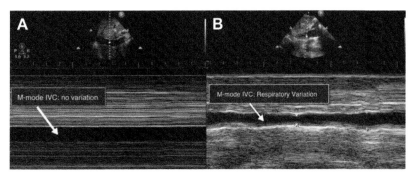

Fig. 16. Inferior vena cava (IVC) in M-mode (*arrows*). Both images are of the proximal IVC (subcostal long-axis view) using M-mode during a respiratory cycle. In (*A*), no respiratory variation is seen, which suggests an elevated right heart pressure (one of the causes can be fluid overload). In (*B*), moderate variation of IVC diameter is seen, likely within the normal range. See text for further discussion on IVC dynamics.

be only 43% accurate when prospectively applied to its own study group. Based on this reappraisal, the investigators offered a simpler approach: an elevated right heart pressure was suggested by an IVC diameter greater than 2.0 cm and a caval index less than 40%.

- *Right heart pressure and the caval index*. Studies have shown an overlap in baseline IVC diameters of subjects with no cardiac disease and those with left and right heart disease. However, the caval index was notably lower in those with right-sided heart disease.[58] This finding suggests that a key influence in caval index is right-sided pressure. Right-sided pressure increases may be elevated in many forms of heart disease, including congestive heart failure (considered a fluid overload states), and pericardial and several pulmonary conditions.[70] IVC plethora itself is not pathognomonic of a single cardiopulmonary disease state or volume status.
- *Evaluation of preload status*. Ultrasound of the IVC does not reflect LV preload status. Volume status assessments with echocardiography should also include an evaluation of LV end-diastolic dimensions.
- *Mechanical ventilation*. In patients undergoing positive pressure ventilation, the IVC will collapse with expiration, rather than inspiration as seen with spontaneously breathing patients. Although the pattern is opposite, the principle of examination for variation with respirations is still the same and can be interpreted in a similar fashion.
- *Pediatrics*. In pediatric emergency medicine studies, IVC indices had moderately good sensitivities but low specificities for gastroenteritis-related dehydration.[57,71] The wide range of sizes in the pediatric age spectrum and patient compliance issues can sometimes make technical measurements of IVC indices difficult. Often the IVC is compared with the aorta for a size reference, and IVC/aorta ratios are commonly measured in children for this reason.[57,71] Note that incidental findings of congenital heart abnormalities are often encountered during emergency echo of children for other indications. Congenital heart abnormality detection is beyond the scope of emergency echocardiography. If the clinician is suspicious of a congenital anomaly, comprehensive pediatric echocardiography is needed for detailed analysis.

Case 5 Conclusion

Based on clinical factors and vital signs alone, this patient appears to be volume depleted. He received volume resuscitation in the ED with clinical improvement. Comprehensive echocardiography was performed on stabilization and, sure enough, this patient was found to have evidence of pulmonary hypertension. The elevated right-sided pressures were likely responsible for his lack of IVC variation despite his dehydrated state.

The bottom line is that, in general, significant IVC diameter respiratory variation usually indicates a hypovolemic state especially when combined with a hyperdynamic and poorly filled heart. However, the presence of a plethoric IVC should not rule out a low volume state, due to the factors previously mentioned. Other causes of elevated right heart pressure should be considered when an IVC diameter greater than 2 cm with less than 40% collapsibility is discovered.[69]

SUMMARY

The responsible and proficient use of emergency echocardiography requires training, knowledge of ultrasound physics, consistent practice in adequate image acquisition, and judicious interpretation. The ACEP *Emergency Ultrasound Guidelines* provides details of minimum training requirements and suggestions for practice-based pathways to training and credentialing in emergency echocardiography. Emergency echocardiography has its limitations and challenges in the emergency setting, but, when used properly, is frequently instrumental and invaluable in improving patient care in the ED.

SUPPLEMENTARY DATA

Supplementary data related to this article can be found online at doi:10.1016/j.emc.2011.08.002.

REFERENCES

1. American College of Emergency Physicians. Emergency ultrasound guidelines. 2008. Available at: http://www.acep.org. Accessed March 28, 2011.
2. Society for Academic Emergency Medicine. Ultrasound position statement. Available at: http://www.saem.org. Accessed March 29, 2011.
3. Labovitz AJ, Noble VE, Bierig M, et al. Focused cardiac ultrasound in the emergent setting: a consensus statement of the American Society of Echocardiography and American College of Emergency Physicians. J Am Soc Echocardiogr 2010;23(12):1225–30.
4. Akhtar S, Theodoro D, Gaspari R, et al. Resident training in emergency ultrasound: consensus recommendations from the 2008 Council of Emergency Medicine Residency Directors Conference. Acad Emerg Med 2009;16(Suppl 2): S32–6.
5. Price S, Via G, Sloth E, et al. Echocardiography practice, training and accreditation in the intensive care: document for the World Interactive Network Focused on Critical Ultrasound (WINFOCUS). Cardiovasc Ultrasound 2008;6:49.
6. Cheitlin MD, Alpert JS, Armstrong WF, et al. ACC/AHA Guidelines for the Clinical Application of Echocardiography. A report of the American College of Cardiology/American Heart Association Task Force on Practice Guidelines (Committee on Clinical Application of Echocardiography). Developed in collaboration with the American Society of Echocardiography. Circulation 1997;95(6):1686–744.
7. Cheitlin MD, Armstrong WF, Aurigemma GP, et al. ACC/AHA/ASE 2003 guideline update for the clinical application of echocardiography: summary article: a report of the American College of Cardiology/American Heart Association Task Force on Practice Guidelines (ACC/AHA/ASE Committee to Update the 1997 Guidelines for the Clinical Application of Echocardiography). Circulation 2003;108(9): 1146–62.
8. Kaul S, Stratienko AA, Pollock SG, et al. Value of two-dimensional echocardiography for determining the basis of hemodynamic compromise in critically ill patients: a prospective study. J Am Soc Echocardiogr 1994;7(6):598–606.
9. Lehmann KG, Johnson AD, Goldberger AL. Mitral valve E point-septal separation as an index of left ventricular function with valvular heart disease. Chest 1983; 83(1):102–8.
10. Massie BM, Schiller NB, Ratshin RA, et al. Mitral-septal separation: new echocardiographic index of left ventricular function. Am J Cardiol 1977;39(7):1008–16.
11. Weekes A, Tassone H, Babcock A, et al. Comparison of serial qualitative and quantitative assessments of caval index and left ventricular systolic function during early fluid resuscitation of hypotensive emergency department patients. Acad Emerg Med 2011;18:912–21.

12. Randazzo MR, Snoey ER, Levitt MA, et al. Accuracy of emergency physician assessment of left ventricular ejection fraction and central venous pressure using echocardiography. Acad Emerg Med 2003;10(9):973–7.
13. Moore CL, Rose GA, Tayal VS, et al. Determination of left ventricular function by emergency physician echocardiography of hypotensive patients. Acad Emerg Med 2002;9(3):186–93.
14. Pershad J, Myers S, Plouman C, et al. Bedside limited echocardiography by the emergency physician is accurate during evaluation of the critically ill patient. Pediatrics 2004;114(6):e667–71.
15. Hollenberg SM. Recognition and treatment of cardiogenic shock. Semin Respir Crit Care Med 2004;25(6):661–71.
16. Nagdev A, Stone MB. Point-of-care ultrasound evaluation of pericardial effusions: Does this patient have cardiac tamponade? Resuscitation 2011;82(6): 671–3.
17. Maggiolini S, Bozzano A, Russo P, et al. Echocardiography-guided pericardiocentesis with probe-mounted needle: report of 53 cases. J Am Soc Echocardiogr 2001;14(8):821–4.
18. Tsang TS, Oh JK, Seward JB. Diagnosis and management of cardiac tamponade in the era of echocardiography. Clin Cardiol 1999;22(7):446–52.
19. Wood KE. Major pulmonary embolism: review of a pathophysiologic approach to the golden hour of hemodynamically significant pulmonary embolism. Chest 2002;121(3):877–905.
20. Toosi MS, Merlino JD, Leeper KV. Prognostic value of the shock index along with transthoracic echocardiography in risk stratification of patients with acute pulmonary embolism. Am J Cardiol 2008;101(5):700–5.
21. Pruszczyk P, Bochowicz A, Torbicki A, et al. Cardiac troponin T monitoring identifies high-risk group of normotensive patients with acute pulmonary embolism. Chest 2003;123(6):1947–52.
22. Fisman DN, Malcolm ID, Ward ME. Echocardiographic detection of pulmonary embolism in transit: implications for institution of thrombolytic therapy. Can J Cardiol 1997;13(7):685–7.
23. Madan A, Schwartz C. Echocardiographic visualization of acute pulmonary embolus and thrombolysis in the ED. Am J Emerg Med 2004;22(4): 294–300.
24. Mansencal N, Redheuil A, Joseph T, et al. Use of transthoracic echocardiography combined with venous ultrasonography in patients with pulmonary embolism. Int J Cardiol 2004;96(1):59–63.
25. Torbicki A, Pruszczyk P. The role of echocardiography in suspected and established PE. Semin Vasc Med 2001;1(2):165–74.
26. Miniati M, Monti S, Pratali L, et al. Value of transthoracic echocardiography in the diagnosis of pulmonary embolism: results of a prospective study in unselected patients. Am J Med 2001;110(7):528–35.
27. Mansencal N, Vieillard-Baron A, Beauchet A, et al. Triage patients with suspected pulmonary embolism in the emergency department using a portable ultrasound device. Echocardiography 2008;25(5):451–6.
28. Kurkciyan I, Meron G, Sterz F, et al. Pulmonary embolism as a cause of cardiac arrest: presentation and outcome. Arch Intern Med 2000;160(10):1529–35.
29. Bova C, Pesavento R, Marchiori A, et al. Risk stratification and outcomes in hemodynamically stable patients with acute pulmonary embolism: a prospective, multicentre, cohort study with three months of follow-up. J Thromb Haemost 2009;7(6): 938–44.

30. Kline JA. Risk stratification and outcomes in hemodynamically stable patients with acute pulmonary embolism: a prospective multicenter, cohort study: a rebuttal. J Thromb Haemost 2009;7(9):1601–2 [author reply: 1602].

31. Kline JA, Steuerwald MT, Marchick MR, et al. Prospective evaluation of right ventricular function and functional status 6 months after acute submassive pulmonary embolism: frequency of persistent or subsequent elevation in estimated pulmonary artery pressure. Chest 2009;136(5):1202–10.

32. American College of Emergency Physicians Clinical Policies Committee, Clinical Policies Committee Subcommittee on Suspected Pulmonary Embolism. Clinical policy: critical issues in the evaluation and management of adult patients presenting with suspected pulmonary embolism. Ann Emerg Med 2003;41(2):257–70.

33. AlMahameed A, Bartholomew JR. Patients with acute pulmonary embolism should have an echocardiogram to guide treatment decisions. Med Clin North Am 2003;87(6):1251–62.

34. Edlow JA. Emergency department management of pulmonary embolism. Emerg Med Clin North Am 2001;19(4):995–1011.

35. Pruszczyk P, Torbicki A, Pacho R, et al. Noninvasive diagnosis of suspected severe pulmonary embolism: transesophageal echocardiography vs spiral CT. Chest 1997;112(3):722–8.

36. Breitkreutz R, Price S, Steiger HV, et al. Focused echocardiographic evaluation in life support and peri-resuscitation of emergency patients: a prospective trial. Resuscitation 2010;81(11):1527–33.

37. Hernandez C, Shuler K, Hannan H, et al. C.A.U.S.E.: Cardiac arrest ultrasound exam—a better approach to managing patients in primary non-arrhythmogenic cardiac arrest. Resuscitation 2008;76(2):198–206.

38. Niendorff DF, Rassias AJ, Palac R, et al. Rapid cardiac ultrasound of inpatients suffering PEA arrest performed by nonexpert sonographers. Resuscitation 2005;67(1):81–7.

39. Price S, Ilper H, Uddin S, et al. Peri-resuscitation echocardiography: training the novice practitioner. Resuscitation 2010;81(11):1534–9.

40. Varriale P, Maldonado JM. Echocardiographic observations during in hospital cardiopulmonary resuscitation. Crit Care Med 1997;25(10):1717–20.

41. ECC Committee, Subcommittees and Task Forces of the American Heart Association. 2005 American Heart Association Guidelines for Cardiopulmonary Resuscitation and Emergency Cardiovascular Care. Circulation 2005;112(Suppl 24): IV1–203.

42. Neumar RW, Otto CW, Link MS, et al. Part 8: adult advanced cardiovascular life support: 2010 American Heart Association Guidelines for Cardiopulmonary Resuscitation and Emergency Cardiovascular Care. Circulation 2010; 122(18 Suppl 3):S729–67.

43. Tayal VS, Beatty MA, Marx JA, et al. FAST (focused assessment with sonography in trauma) accurate for cardiac and intraperitoneal injury in penetrating anterior chest trauma. J Ultrasound Med 2004;23(4):467–72.

44. Tayal VS, Kline JA. Emergency echocardiography to detect pericardial effusion in patients in PEA and near-PEA states. Resuscitation 2003;59(3):315–8.

45. Jones AE, Tayal VS, Kline JA. Focused training of emergency medicine residents in goal-directed echocardiography: a prospective study. Acad Emerg Med 2003; 10(10):1054–8.

46. Breitkreutz R, Walcher F, Seeger FH. Focused echocardiographic evaluation in resuscitation management: concept of an advanced life support-conformed algorithm. Crit Care Med 2007;35(Suppl 5):S150–61.

47. Blaivas M, Fox JC. Outcome in cardiac arrest patients found to have cardiac standstill on the bedside emergency department echocardiogram. Acad Emerg Med 2001;8(6):616–21.
48. Salen P, O'Connor R, Sierzenski P, et al. Can cardiac sonography and capnography be used independently and in combination to predict resuscitation outcomes? Acad Emerg Med 2001;8(6):610–5.
49. Kan H, Failinger CF, Fang Q, et al. Reversible myocardial dysfunction in sepsis and ischemia. Crit Care Med 2005;33(12):2845–7.
50. Machiels JP, Dive A, Donckier J, et al. Reversible myocardial dysfunction in a patient with alcoholic ketoacidosis: a role for hypophosphatemia. Am J Emerg Med 1998;16(4):371–3.
51. Ruiz Bailen M. Reversible myocardial dysfunction in critically ill, noncardiac patients: a review. Crit Care Med 2002;30(6):1280–90.
52. Braunwald E, Kloner RA. The stunned myocardium: prolonged, postischemic ventricular dysfunction. Circulation 1982;66(6):1146–9.
53. Laurent I, Monchi M, Chiche JD, et al. Reversible myocardial dysfunction in survivors of out-of-hospital cardiac arrest. J Am Coll Cardiol 2002;40(12):2110–6.
54. Kleinman ME, Chameides L, Schexnayder SM, et al. Part 14: pediatric advanced life support: 2010 American Heart Association Guidelines for Cardiopulmonary Resuscitation and Emergency Cardiovascular Care. Circulation 2010;122 (18 Suppl 3):S876–908.
55. Tsung JW, Blaivas M. Feasibility of correlating the pulse check with focused point-of-care echocardiography during pediatric cardiac arrest: a case series. Resuscitation 2008;77(2):264–9.
56. McGee S, Abernethy WB 3rd, Simel DL. The rational clinical examination. Is this patient hypovolemic? JAMA 1999;281(11):1022–9.
57. Chen L, Hsiao A, Langhan M, et al. Use of bedside ultrasound to assess degree of dehydration in children with gastroenteritis. Acad Emerg Med 2010;17(10):1042–7.
58. Moreno FL, Hagan AD, Holmen JR, et al. Evaluation of size and dynamics of the inferior vena cava as an index of right-sided cardiac function. Am J Cardiol 1984; 53(4):579–85.
59. Barbier C, Loubieres Y, Schmit C, et al. Respiratory changes in inferior vena cava diameter are helpful in predicting fluid responsiveness in ventilated septic patients. Intensive Care Med 2004;30(9):1740–6.
60. Feissel M, Michard F, Faller JP, et al. The respiratory variation in inferior vena cava diameter as a guide to fluid therapy. Intensive Care Med 2004;30(9):1834–7.
61. Fields JM, Lee PA, Jenq KY, et al. The interrater reliability of inferior vena cava ultrasound by bedside clinician sonographers in emergency department patients. Acad Emerg Med 2011;18(1):98–101.
62. Mintz GS, Kotler MN, Parry WR, et al. Real-time inferior vena caval ultrasonography: normal and abnormal findings and its use in assessing right-heart function. Circulation 1981;64(5):1018–25.
63. Bendjelid K, Romand JA, Walder B, et al. Correlation between measured inferior vena cava diameter and right atrial pressure depends on the echocardiographic method used in patients who are mechanically ventilated. J Am Soc Echocardiogr 2002;15(9):944–9.
64. Carr BG, Dean AJ, Everett WW, et al. Intensivist bedside ultrasound (INBU) for volume assessment in the intensive care unit: a pilot study. J Trauma 2007; 63(3):495–500 [discussion: 500–2].
65. Lyon M, Blaivas M, Brannam L. Sonographic measurement of the inferior vena cava as a marker of blood loss. Am J Emerg Med 2005;23(1):45–50.

66. Krause I, Birk E, Davidovits M, et al. Inferior vena cava diameter: a useful method for estimation of fluid status in children on haemodialysis. Nephrol Dial Transplant 2001;16(6):1203–6.

67. Kircher BJ, Himelman RB, Schiller NB. Noninvasive estimation of right atrial pressure from the inspiratory collapse of the inferior vena cava. Am J Cardiol 1990; 66(4):493–6.

68. Nagdev AD, Merchant RC, Tirado-Gonzalez A, et al. Emergency department bedside ultrasonographic measurement of the caval index for noninvasive determination of low central venous pressure. Ann Emerg Med 2010;55(3):290–5.

69. Brennan JM, Blair JE, Goonewardena S, et al. Reappraisal of the use of inferior vena cava for estimating right atrial pressure. J Am Soc Echocardiogr 2007; 20(7):857–61.

70. Blehar DJ, Dickman E, Gaspari R. Identification of congestive heart failure via respiratory variation of inferior vena cava diameter. Am J Emerg Med 2009; 27(1):71–5.

71. Levine AC, Shah SP, Umulisa I, et al. Ultrasound assessment of severe dehydration in children with diarrhea and vomiting. Acad Emerg Med 2010;17(10): 1035–41.

Aortic Emergencies

Kathleen Wittels, MD[a,b],*

KEYWORDS

- Aortic dissection • Abdominal aortic aneurysm
- Thoracic aortic aneurysm

Patients with aortic emergencies are some of the highest acuity patients that the Emergency Medicine (EM) physician encounters. These emergencies are divided into 2 primary groups: those related to aortic dissection and those related to an abdominal aortic aneurysm (AAA). Thoracic aortic aneurysms without dissection comprise a smaller subset of patients with aortic emergencies. Because there are varying presenting complaints, these diagnoses can be challenging to make, and a missed diagnosis often leads to significant morbidity and mortality. This article discusses the clinical presentations, available diagnostic tools, and treatment considerations of aortic dissection, AAA, and thoracic aortic aneurysm.

AORTIC DISSECTION
Causes and Risk Factors

Acute aortic dissection occurs when there is a tear in the aortic intima, resulting in separation between the aortic intima and the aortic media. Blood flows into this space, creating the false lumen. The initial tear may propagate proximally and/or distally and affect any arteries branching from the aorta, resulting in varied clinical presentations. Because of this, as well as the relative infrequency of the diagnosis, aortic dissection is a diagnosis that can be challenging for the emergency physician.

Several risk factors have been associated with aortic dissection.[1] These include:

- Hypertension
- Stimulant use
- Trauma
- Genetic conditions including Marfan syndrome, Ehlers-Danlos syndrome, bicuspid aortic valve
- Inflammatory vasculitides including Takayesu arteritis, giant cell arteritis, and Behçet arteritis

There is no funding support for this article, and the author has nothing to disclose.
[a] Harvard Medical School, USA
[b] Department of Emergency Medicine, Brigham and Women's Hospital, 75 Francis Street, Neville House, Boston, MA 02115, USA
* Department of Emergency Medicine, Brigham and Women's Hospital, 75 Francis Street, Neville House, Boston, MA 02115.
E-mail address: kwittels@partners.org

- Family history of aortic disease
- History of recent aortic manipulation
- History of known thoracic aortic aneurysm.

Clinical Presentation

The most common presenting symptoms of an aortic dissection are chest pain and/or back pain.[2] Chest pain that is sudden in onset, tearing in quality, or of severe intensity suggests an aortic dissection.[3] In addition to chest and/or back pain, hypertension is a common finding at the time of presentation and is seen in greater than two-thirds of patients.[2] Additional signs and symptoms that may be present include:

- Abdominal pain
- Migrating pain
- Pulse deficit
- Focal neurologic deficit
- Diastolic murmur (aortic insufficiency)
- Flank pain.

Although a pulse discrepancy between extremities is classically associated with aortic dissection, this sign has been found to have a sensitivity of only 31%. When it is present, though, it strongly suggests aortic dissection. Focal neurologic complaints also suggest dissection when present, but the lack of neurologic deficits does not help to exclude the diagnosis.[3]

Classification

Aortic dissections are classified by their anatomic location. Aortic dissections of the ascending aorta are twice as common as those involving the descending aorta. There are 2 different classification systems for aortic dissections (**Fig. 1**). One classification system is the Debakey system, which divides aortic dissections into 3 types based on the origin of the intimal tear:

- Type I: originates in the ascending aorta and involves both the ascending and the descending aorta
- Type II: originates in and involves only the ascending aorta
- Type III: originates in and involves only the descending aorta.

The Stanford system divides aortic dissections into 2 groups based on involvement of the ascending aorta, correlating with the likely treatment course:

- Type A (proximal): involves the ascending aorta with or without involvement of the descending aorta (usually surgical management)
- Type B (distal): involves only the descending aorta (usually medical management).

Diagnostic Modalities

Chest radiography
Chest radiography is easily obtained in the emergency department and is often one of the first tests available in the evaluation of a patient with aortic dissection. The presence of a widened mediastinum (>8 cm) is concerning for dissection (**Fig. 2**). Other findings include an abnormal aortic contour, the calcium sign (separation of calcific intima from outer aortic soft tissue), left pleural effusion, and depression of the left mainstem bronchus. Abnormalities on chest radiography are present in greater than 80% of patients with aortic dissection.[4]

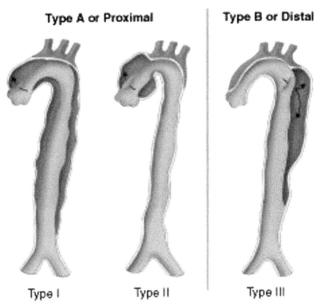

Type A or Proximal   **Type B or Distal**

Type I   Type II   Type III

Fig. 1. Classification of aortic dissection by the Stanford system (labels at top) and Debakey system (labels at bottom). (*From* Isselbacher EM. Diseases of the aorta. In: Braunwald E, Zipes DP, Libby P, et al, editors. Braunwald's heart disease: a textbook of cardiovascular medicine. 7th edition. Philadelphia: Saunders; 2004. p. 1416; with permission.)

Computed tomography imaging

Computed tomography (CT) scans are widely available, and CT with angiography (CTA) has become the imaging modality of choice for the evaluation of stable patients with acute aortic dissection. Advantages of CT scans include the ability to evaluate the location of the dissection flap and to aid in operative planning for ascending aortic dissections. **Fig. 3** illustrates a Stanford type A dissection. The disadvantage of the CTA is that it requires a contrast bolus, which is not ideal for patients with renal

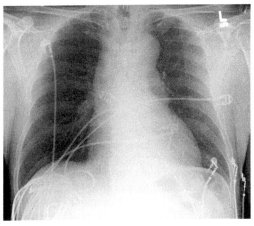

Fig. 2. A widened mediastinum in a patient with aortic dissection.

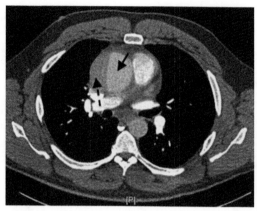

Fig. 3. Axial image from a chest CT scan showing an aortic dissection involving the ascending aorta. Both the true lumen (*solid arrow*) and false lumen (*dashed arrow*) are visible.

insufficiency. In addition, unstable patients may not be able to leave the emergency department bay for the study and other modalities must be considered.

Transesophageal echocardiography

Transesophageal echocardiography (TEE) can be performed at the bedside, which makes it an ideal study for the evaluation of unstable patients. Although extremely sensitive and specific in experienced hands, TEE is operator dependent. It has the advantage compared with CT imaging of being able to evaluate the aortic root to assess for acute aortic insufficiency associated with the dissection.

Other imaging modalities

Magnetic resonance imaging (MRI) is sensitive for the identification of an aortic dissection but is less often used to make the diagnosis. Many patients with suspected aortic dissection are not stable enough for MRI, and MRI availability is variable. The advantages associated with MRI are the lack of radiation and the ability of MRI to detail the location and extension of the dissection.

Transthoracic echocardiography (TTE) may be able to visualize an aortic dissection, but TTE is not sensitive for this diagnosis and should not be used on its own to rule out the disease process. TTE is often used in combination with TEE for better visualization of the aortic arch (there is a blind spot in the distal portion of the aortic arch on TEE). **Fig. 4** depict an image obtained with TTE correlating with the CT image in **Fig. 3**.

Laboratory studies

There is no universally accepted biomarker or assay to diagnose or rule out aortic dissection. The D dimer assay has been suggested as an option to rule out low-risk patients for aortic dissection, much as it is used to rule out low-risk patients for pulmonary embolism. Multiple studies have shown increased D dimer levels in patients with aortic dissection.[5–8] Meta-analyses have shown high sensitivity of the D dimer in identifying patients with aortic dissection, ranging from 94% to 97%, with lower specificity.[9,10] A subset of patients with aortic dissection who have a thrombus in the false lumen and a short dissection length have been noted to have negative D dimers.[11] Although it is appealing to avoid the need for advanced imaging studies to exclude the

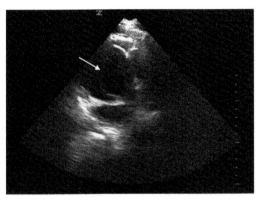

Fig. 4. Transthoracic ultrasound image of the same patient as in **Fig. 3**. The arrowhead points to the dissection flap.

diagnosis of aortic dissection, it is unclear at this time whether the D dimer can do this for the diagnosis of aortic dissection.

Decision rules

One of the challenges in evaluating patients for aortic dissection is that there have been no well-established decision rules to help categorize patients as low risk for aortic the way the Wells criteria do for the evaluation of patients with suspected pulmonary embolism. In 2010, a guideline was published for the evaluation and treatment of patients with thoracic aortic disease.[1] Within this guideline, the investigators present a risk-assessment tool to identify patients as low, moderate, or high risk for aortic dissection based on the presence of high-risk conditions, high-risk pain features, and high-risk examination features. Within the pathway, patients classified as moderate or high risk have aortic imaging.

Recently, this risk-assessment tool was applied to the International Registry of Acute Aortic Dissection and was found to have a sensitivity greater than 95%.[12] However, 4.3% of patients in this registry with known aortic dissection would have been classified as low risk and potentially would have been missed. It is also unclear how the tool will perform in an undifferentiated patient population with suspected aortic dissection. Prospective investigation may shed further light on the general applicability of this tool.

Treatment

Medical

All patients with aortic dissections require aggressive blood pressure and heart rate control to limit shear force on the aorta, which can lead to propagation of the dissection. The target systolic blood pressure is 100 to 120 mm Hg and goal heart rate is 60 beats per minute.[13] There are several classes of medications that are used to reach these targets.

β-Blockers β-Blockers are first-line therapy for aortic dissection because of their combined effects in lowering both blood pressure and heart rate. Esmolol is a good choice given that it is a short-acting agent and can be titrated to effect (starting dose 500 μg/kg bolus, followed by infusion at 50 μg/kg/min; rebolus and increase drip rate by 50 μg/kg/min every 4 minutes until target vital signs have been reached). If esmolol is not available, labetolol is an alternative choice.

Nitroprusside Once the heart rate has been well controlled, vasodilators such as nitro-prusside can be added if additional blood pressure reduction is needed. Nitroprusside acts by reducing both preload and afterload. It is important that nitroprusside is only added after β-blockers because it can cause reflex tachycardia when used independently, thereby increasing aortic stress and potentially resulting in a worsening dissection. Nitroprusside is given as a continuous infusion at a rate of 0.5 to 3 μg/kg/min. Higher doses should be avoided because of the risk of cyanide toxicity.

Calcium channel blockers Although calcium channel blockers such as verapamil or diltiazem are not commonly used in the medical management of aortic dissection, they can be substituted if the patient has a contraindication to β-blocker administration.

Surgical
Most patients with an aortic dissection involving the ascending aorta require surgical intervention. If cardiac surgery is not available at the diagnostic center, patients require emergent transfer to a tertiary care hospital. While awaiting surgical intervention or transfer, it is crucial to continue aggressive medical management. Some patients with a descending aortic dissection are also considered for surgical intervention, including those with aortic rupture or evidence of visceral or limb ischemia. Older patients (>70 years) and those with preoperative shock have been shown to have higher surgical mortality.[14]

Other interventions
Endovascular stenting is a newer intervention used in the treatment of aortic dissection, particularly as an alternative to surgery for patients with Stanford type B aortic dissections with evidence of limb or visceral ischemia. Its feasibility was first studied in the 1990s.[15,16] Refractory or recurrent pain and/or refractory hypertension are considered poor prognostic indicators for survival in patients with descending aortic dissections. Investigators of the International Registry of Acute Aortic Dissection (IRAD) studied this population and showed that these patients have lower mortalities with endovascular intervention compared with medical management alone.[17] For patients with ruptured descending thoracic aortic aneurysms, a recent meta-analysis showed lower 30-day mortality for patients treated with an endovascular approach versus open surgery (19% vs 33%).[18]

An alternative to endovascular stenting, aortic fenestration may help to restore perfusion to patients with evidence of end-organ injury. With this procedure, communication is established between the true and false lumens of the aorta to allow blood flow to arteries originating from the false lumen. Surgical aortic fenestration has been suggested as an alternative option to aortic replacement as well as in the case of contraindicated or failed endovascular stenting.[16,19,20]

AAA
Causes and Risk Factors

A ruptured AAA is a catastrophic cardiovascular condition with high morbidity and mortality.

Risk factors for AAA include

- Age greater than 60 years
- Male sex
- Tobacco use
- Family history of AAA
- History of heart disease or peripheral vascular disease
- Hypertension.

Clinical Presentation

Unruptured aneurysms are often asymptomatic, resulting in a diagnosis that is challenging to make. Multiple studies have evaluated the mortality benefit and cost-effectiveness of routine screening for AAA, with conflicting results.[21–28] The US Preventive Services Task Force recommends screening men aged 65 to 75 years with a history of smoking. The task force recommends against screening men without a smoking history or women because of the low incidence of AAA in these groups.[29]

Patients with a ruptured AAA usually present with severe abdominal pain. Other symptoms that may also be present include back or flank pain, hypotension, and syncope. The triad of syncope, abdominal pain, and hypotension is highly suggestive of a vascular catastrophe. A patient with a history of a prior AAA presenting with a catastrophic gastrointestinal bleed suggests the development of an aortoenteric fistula.

Physical examination can be limited for the diagnosis of an unruptured AAA. A pulsatile abdominal mass may be palpable. This finding increases in sensitivity with enlarging aneurysm size as well as with smaller abdominal girth.[30,31] One study has noted that the sensitivity of abdominal palpation increases from 29% for AAAs between 3.0 and 3.9 cm, to 50% for AAAs between 4.0 and 4.9 cm, to 76% for AAAs 5.0 cm or greater.[30] Once the AAA ruptures, abdominal tenderness is common. However, in the absence of hemodynamic instability, the diagnosis can remain challenging, which was shown in a review of a group of patients with ruptured AAA presenting to internists. In 61% of cases, the diagnosis was initially missed and only identified once there was hemodynamic compromise.[32]

Diagnostic Modalities

Ultrasonography is one of the most readily available modalities for the evaluation of patients with suspected AAA. It has a high sensitivity and specificity, making it an ideal test for both diagnosing and following an AAA. A normal-diameter aorta is defined as being smaller than 3.0 cm. When evaluating the aorta with ultrasound, it is important to obtain measurements at multiple levels and to include both axial and longitudinal views.

Although traditionally performed by ultrasound technicians and interpreted by radiologists, there have been multiple studies evaluating the use of bedside ultrasound by the emergency physician. Results suggest that, with minimal training, emergency physicians can identify AAAs with high sensitivity and specificity.[33,34] Advantages of performing ultrasound by emergency physicians for the diagnosis of AAA include the ability to make a rapid diagnosis at the patient's bedside as well as the ability to make the diagnosis in settings with limited ultrasound technician and radiology support. **Fig. 5** illustrates an AAA identified with bedside ultrasound in the emergency department.

CT scan imaging is an alternative to ultrasonography for the diagnosis of AAA. CT scans are limited in that they can only be performed in stable patients, but there are advantages to this modality. CT scans can characterize and confirm the extent of the lesion, which is helpful for operative planning. In addition, unlike ultrasound, CT scans are less operator dependent. MRI is not commonly used in the initial work-up and diagnosis of AAA, but an AAA may be seen on an abdominal MRI obtained for other reasons.

Treatment

Treatment of an AAA depends on its size as well as whether or not it is ruptured. Unruptured AAAs identified in asymptomatic patients may be monitored for

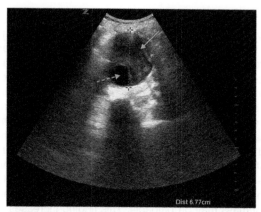

Fig. 5. Transverse view of the abdominal aorta obtained with bedside ultrasound. Anteroposterior measurement of the aorta shows a 6.77-cm aneurysm. Both the intramural thrombus (*solid arrow*) and the aorta lumen (*dashed arrow*) are depicted.

progression. Symptomatic and ruptured aneurysms require surgical intervention. Once an asymptomatic aneurysm is greater than 5 cm, operative repair is generally recommended.[35] Based on the law of Laplace (tension is proportional to pressure and radius), the rate of expansion increases as the lumen size increases. Beyond 5 cm, the risk of rupture generally exceeds that of operative risk.

Treatment of patients with unruptured AAAs smaller than 5 cm centers around risk factor modification and monitoring for expansion of the aneurysm. Smoking cessation should be encouraged. Initiation of β-blocker therapy is also recommended in patients with AAAs. Although studies are limited, β-blockers have been shown to reduce the rate of aneurysm expansion, and the American College of Cardiology and American Heart Association recommend initiation of β-blockers in patients with AAAs.[36]

The initial treatment of a patient with a ruptured AAA is focused on hemodynamic stabilization. Multiple large-bore intravenous lines should be placed, and infusion of crystalloid should begin immediately in hypotensive patients. Uncrossmatched packed red blood cells can be initiated and then switched to crossmatched packed red blood cells when available. Platelets and fresh frozen plasma will likely be needed, given the large-volume transfusions that occur with these patients. It is important to know the capabilities of the blood bank in the practice setting. If there are limited blood products available, rapid patient transfer becomes more critical.

There is no consensus on specific vital sign goals of resuscitation in hypotensive patients with ruptured AAAs. Instead, the focus is to resuscitate to vital organ function. Follow mental status and urine output to assess brain and kidney function. Serial electrocardiograms assessing for evidence of cardiac ischemia may be useful. Over-resuscitation may lead to possible clot disruption. There is also a concern for dilution of clotting factors if resuscitation is limited to crystalloid and packed red blood cells.

When the diagnosis of a ruptured AAA is made, a vascular surgeon should be consulted immediately. Depending on operative capabilities of the treating institution, patients with ruptured AAAs may require emergent transfer to tertiary care centers if they can be stabilized for transport. There are 2 different options for the repair of a ruptured AAA: open versus endovascular repair. Multiple studies have compared the mortalities of the 2 options. The endovascular approach has been shown to have a lower short-term mortality, but this advantage is lost over time because of the incidence of graft failure.[37–40]

THORACIC AORTIC ANEURYSM
Causes and Risk Factors

Thoracic aortic aneurysms (TAAs) are less common than AAAs. They are described based on their location within the thoracic aorta: the aortic root, the ascending thoracic aorta, the aortic arch, or the descending thoracic aorta.[41] Aneurysms may also extend into the abdominal aorta and are then called thoracoabdominal aneurysms. Risk factors for TAAs are similar to those for AAAs.

Clinical Presentation

As with AAAs, TAAs are often asymptomatic until they rupture. The most common presenting symptom of rupture is pain in the chest or back. Additional symptoms are determined by the location and size of the aneurysm. Aortic root and ascending TAAs can cause aortic insufficiency, resulting in heart failure. They can also obstruct the superior vena cava if they are large, resulting in distended neck veins on examination. TAAs can cause hoarseness from stretching of the recurrent laryngeal nerves, and descending TAAs can compress the trachea, resulting in respiratory symptoms such as wheezing, cough, or dyspnea. Compression of the esophagus causes dysphagia.[41]

Diagnostic Modalities

TAAs are often first suspected after chest radiography is obtained for another indication. Findings include a widened mediastinum, tracheal deviation, and enlargement of the aortic knob. However, normal chest radiography does not rule out a TAA. Similarly to the work-up for aortic dissections, CT scan imaging is the most common modality used. Echocardiography is a good alternative if a CT scan cannot be obtained, and has the functional advantage of being able to assess the aortic valve function. Although MRI provides detailed characterization of TAAs, it is less commonly used in the work-up of a TAA.

Treatment

Patients with ruptured TAAs require resuscitation in the same manner as those with ruptured AAAs, as well as emergent cardiothoracic surgical consultation. Asymptomatic patients with TAAs may be monitored with serial imaging for aneurysm growth. β-Blockers are recommended in an attempt to slow aneurysm growth. The decision for operative intervention in asymptomatic patients with TAA is determined by the aneurysm size and rate of expansion, similarly to the approach of AAAs. The annual risk of TAA rupture has been shown to increase from 2% for aneurysms less than 5 cm, to 3% for those 5 cm to 5.9 cm, to 7% for those greater than 6 cm.[42] Studies evaluating the risk of rupture in untreated TAAs have led to a recommendation that ascending TAAs greater than 5.5 cm and descending TAAs greater than 6.5 cm should receive intervention.[43,44] Patients with Marfan syndrome are considered for earlier intervention because of the higher risk of rupture or dissection.

REFERENCES

1. Hiratzka LF, Bakris GL, Beckman JA, et al. 2010 ACCF/AHA/AATS/ACR/ASA/SCA/SCAI/SIR/STS/SVM guidelines for the diagnosis and management of patients with thoracic aortic disease: a report of the American College of Cardiology Foundation/American Heart Association Task Force on Practice Guidelines, American Association for Thoracic Surgery, American College of Radiology, American Stroke Association, Society of Cardiovascular Anesthesiologists,

Society for Cardiovascular Angiography and Interventions, Society of Interventional Radiology, Society of Thoracic Surgeons, and Society for Vascular Medicine. Circulation 2010;121(13):e266–369.

2. Suzuki T, Mehta RH, Ince H, et al. Clinical profiles and outcomes of acute type B aortic dissection in the current era: lessons from the International Registry of Aortic Dissection (IRAD). Circulation 2003;108(Suppl 1):II312–7.

3. Klompas M. Does this patient have an acute thoracic aortic dissection? JAMA 2002;287(17):2262–72.

4. Braverman AC. Acute aortic dissection: clinician update. Circulation 2010;122(2): 184–8.

5. Eggebrecht H, Naber CK, Bruch C, et al. Value of plasma fibrin D-dimers for detection of acute aortic dissection. J Am Coll Cardiol 2004;44(4):804–9.

6. Perez A, Abbet P, Drescher MJ. D-Dimers in the emergency department evaluation of aortic dissection. Acad Emerg Med 2004;11(4):397–400.

7. Weber T, Hogler S, Auer J, et al. D-Dimer in acute aortic dissection. Chest 2003; 123(5):1375–8.

8. Suzuki T, Distante A, Zizza A, et al. Diagnosis of acute aortic dissection by D-dimer: the International Registry of Acute Aortic Dissection Substudy on Biomarkers (IRAD-Bio) experience. Circulation 2009;119(20):2702–7.

9. Sodeck G, Domanovits H, Schillinger M, et al. D-Dimer in ruling out acute aortic dissection: a systematic review and prospective cohort study. Eur Heart J 2007;28(24):3067–75.

10. Marill KA. Serum D-dimer is a sensitive test for the detection of acute aortic dissection: a pooled meta-analysis. J Emerg Med 2008;34(4):367–76.

11. Hazui H, Nishimoto M, Hoshiga M, et al. Young adult patients with short dissection length and thrombosed false lumen without ulcer-like projections are liable to have false-negative results of D-dimer testing for acute aortic dissection based on a study of 113 cases. Circ J 2006;70(12):1598–601.

12. Rogers AM, Hermann LK, Booher AM, et al. Sensitivity of the aortic dissection detection risk score, a novel guideline-based tool for identification of acute aortic dissection at initial presentation: results from the International Registry of Acute Aortic Dissection. Circulation 2011;123(20):2213–8.

13. Tsai TT, Nienaber CA, Eagle KA. Acute aortic syndromes. Circulation 2005; 112(24):3802–13.

14. Trimarchi S, Nienaber CA, Rampoldi V, et al. Role and results of surgery in acute type B aortic dissection: insights from the International Registry of Acute Aortic Dissection (IRAD). Circulation 2006;114(Suppl 1):I357–64.

15. Dake MD, Kato N, Mitchell RS, et al. Endovascular stent-graft placement for the treatment of acute aortic dissection. N Engl J Med 1999;340(20):1546–52.

16. Nienaber CA, Fattori R, Lund G, et al. Nonsurgical reconstruction of thoracic aortic dissection by stent-graft placement. N Engl J Med 1999;340(20): 1539–45.

17. Trimarchi S, Eagle KA, Nienaber CA, et al. Importance of refractory pain and hypertension in acute type B aortic dissection: insights from the International Registry of Acute Aortic Dissection (IRAD). Circulation 2010;122(13):1283–9.

18. Jonker FH, Trimarchi S, Verhagen HJ, et al. Meta-analysis of open versus endovascular repair for ruptured descending thoracic aortic aneurysm. J Vasc Surg 2010;51(4):1026–32, 1032.e1–e2.

19. Pradhan S, Elefteriades JA, Sumpio BE. Utility of the aortic fenestration technique in the management of acute aortic dissections. Ann Thorac Cardiovasc Surg 2007;13(5):296–300.

20. Trimarchi S, Jonker FH, Muhs BE, et al. Long-term outcomes of surgical aortic fenestration for complicated acute type B aortic dissections. J Vasc Surg 2010; 52(2):261–6.

21. Lindholt JS, Juul S, Fasting H, et al. Screening for abdominal aortic aneurysms: single centre randomised controlled trial. BMJ 2005;330(7494):750.

22. Buxton MJ. Screening for abdominal aortic aneurysm. BMJ 2009;338:b2185.

23. Ehlers L, Overvad K, Sorensen J, et al. Analysis of cost effectiveness of screening Danish men aged 65 for abdominal aortic aneurysm. BMJ 2009;338:b2243.

24. Thompson SG, Ashton HA, Gao L, et al. Screening men for abdominal aortic aneurysm: 10 year mortality and cost effectiveness results from the randomised Multicentre Aneurysm Screening Study. BMJ 2009;338:b2307.

25. Ashton HA, Buxton MJ, Day NE, et al. The Multicentre Aneurysm Screening Study (MASS) into the effect of abdominal aortic aneurysm screening on mortality in men: a randomised controlled trial. Lancet 2002;360(9345):1531–9.

26. Cosford PA, Leng GC. Screening for abdominal aortic aneurysm. Cochrane Database Syst Rev 2007;2:CD002945.

27. Fleming C, Whitlock EP, Beil TL, et al. Screening for abdominal aortic aneurysm: a best-evidence systematic review for the U.S. Preventive Services Task Force. Ann Intern Med 2005;142(3):203–11.

28. Lindholt JS, Sorensen J, Sogaard R, et al. Long-term benefit and cost-effectiveness analysis of screening for abdominal aortic aneurysms from a randomized controlled trial. Br J Surg 2010;97(6):826–34.

29. Screening for abdominal aortic aneurysm: recommendation statement. Ann Intern Med 2005;142(3):198–202.

30. Lederle FA, Simel DL. The rational clinical examination. Does this patient have abdominal aortic aneurysm? JAMA 1999;281(1):77–82.

31. Fink HA, Lederle FA, Roth CS, et al. The accuracy of physical examination to detect abdominal aortic aneurysm. Arch Intern Med 2000;160(6):833–6.

32. Lederle FA, Parenti CM, Chute EP. Ruptured abdominal aortic aneurysm: the internist as diagnostician. Am J Med 1994;96(2):163–7.

33. Kuhn M, Bonnin RL, Davey MJ, et al. Emergency department ultrasound scanning for abdominal aortic aneurysm: accessible, accurate, and advantageous. Ann Emerg Med 2000;36(3):219–23.

34. Tayal VS, Graf CD, Gibbs MA. Prospective study of accuracy and outcome of emergency ultrasound for abdominal aortic aneurysm over two years. Acad Emerg Med 2003;10(8):867–71.

35. Ernst CB. Abdominal aortic aneurysm. N Engl J Med 1993;328(16):1167–72.

36. Hirsch AT, Haskal ZJ, Hertzer NR, et al. ACC/AHA 2005 practice guidelines for the management of patients with peripheral arterial disease (lower extremity, renal, mesenteric, and abdominal aortic): a collaborative report from the American Association for Vascular Surgery/Society for Vascular Surgery, Society for Cardiovascular Angiography and Interventions, Society for Vascular Medicine and Biology, Society of Interventional Radiology, and the ACC/AHA Task Force on Practice Guidelines (Writing Committee to Develop Guidelines for the Management of Patients With Peripheral Arterial Disease): endorsed by the American Association of Cardiovascular and Pulmonary Rehabilitation; National Heart, Lung, and Blood Institute; Society for Vascular Nursing; TransAtlantic Inter-Society Consensus; and Vascular Disease Foundation. Circulation 2006;113(11):e463–654.

37. Schermerhorn ML, O'Malley AJ, Jhaveri A, et al. Endovascular vs. open repair of abdominal aortic aneurysms in the Medicare population. N Engl J Med 2008; 358(5):464–74.

38. Lederle FA, Freischlag JA, Kyriakides TC, et al. Outcomes following endovascular vs open repair of abdominal aortic aneurysm: a randomized trial. JAMA 2009; 302(14):1535–42.

39. Greenhalgh RM, Brown LC, Powell JT, et al. Endovascular versus open repair of abdominal aortic aneurysm. N Engl J Med 2010;362(20):1863–71.

40. De Bruin JL, Baas AF, Buth J, et al. Long-term outcome of open or endovascular repair of abdominal aortic aneurysm. N Engl J Med 2010;362(20):1881–9.

41. Isselbacher EM. Thoracic and abdominal aortic aneurysms. Circulation 2005; 111(6):816–28.

42. Davies RR, Goldstein LJ, Coady MA, et al. Yearly rupture or dissection rates for thoracic aortic aneurysms: simple prediction based on size. Ann Thorac Surg 2002;73(1):17–27 [discussion: 27–8].

43. Coady MA, Rizzo JA, Hammond GL, et al. Surgical intervention criteria for thoracic aortic aneurysms: a study of growth rates and complications. Ann Thorac Surg 1999;67(6):1922–6 [discussion: 1953–8].

44. Elefteriades JA. Natural history of thoracic aortic aneurysms: indications for surgery, and surgical versus nonsurgical risks. Ann Thorac Surg 2002;74(5): S1877–80 [discussion: S1892–8].

Diagnosis and Management of Valvular Heart Disease in Emergency Medicine

Richard S. Chen, MD, MBA[a], Matthew J. Bivens, MD[a],
Shamai A. Grossman, MD, MS[b,c],*

KEYWORDS

- Heart murmur • Mechanical valve • Endocarditis
- Aortic stenosis • Mitral regurgitation

A popular saying holds that if one can hear a heart murmur in the middle of a loud and busy emergency department, then by definition the murmur is significant. Whether or not this is actually true, it does capture the frustration emergency physicians feel when trying to diagnose or manage valvular pathologic conditions with familiar yet limited tools, such as the stethoscope, chest radiograph, bedside ultrasound, and electrocardiogram (ECG). Sometimes the emergency physician makes a first diagnosis of a problematic heart valve by noting a previously unmentioned murmur on examination. At other times, patients present to the emergency department (ED) with known valvular disease. Valvular pathologic conditions may be at the very root of the patient's chief complaint, for example, in aortic stenosis causing syncope or acute left-sided valve failure leading to hemodynamic collapse. More often, a valvular pathologic condition is a chronic, sideline issue that, nevertheless, needs to be taken into account when managing patient's other medical needs.

The authors have nothing to disclose.

[a] Harvard-Affiliated Emergency Medicine Residency, Department of Emergency Medicine, Beth Israel Deaconess Medical Center, One Deaconess Road, West Campus Clinical Center, Boston, MA 02215, USA

[b] Clinical Decision Unit and Cardiac Emergency Center, Beth Israel Deaconess Medical Center, Boston, MA, USA

[c] Department of Emergency Medicine, Beth Israel Deaconess Medical Center, Harvard Medical School, One Deaconess Road, Boston, MA 02215, USA

* Corresponding author. Department of Emergency Medicine, Beth Israel Deaconess Medical Center, Harvard Medical School, One Deaconess Road, Boston, MA 02215.
E-mail address: sgrossma@bidmc.harvard.edu

This article focuses on the valve-related issues the emergency physician will face, from the trauma patient with a mechanical valve who may need his or her anticoagulation reversed to the febrile patient with a new murmur.

THE DISORDERED HEART VALVE
Epidemiology and Pathophysiology

In the developing world, rheumatic fever remains an important cause of valvular disease. But elsewhere, antibiotics for streptococcal infections have greatly reduced rheumatic heart disease prevalence, making valvular disease in the medically privileged nations generally either an inherited or congenital issue (ie, related to Marfan-associated dissection or bicuspid aortic valve), or, more often, a result of age-associated wear and tear.

Prosthetic valves
As the population ages, we are more and more likely to encounter patients with valvular disease and the sequela related to repair and treatment of this disease. Valvular disease now accounts for up to 20% of all cardiac surgeries in the United States.[1] There are approximately 40,000 replacement valve operations performed each year in the United States, with more than 80 different types of artificial valves, from mechanical to bioprosthetic.[2,3]

Aortic stenosis
Left-sided valvular lesions are the most commonly encountered in clinical practice, in part because right-sided valvular lesions have a prolonged latent asymptomatic period.[4] In turn, aortic stenosis is the most common of all valvular diseases in the developed world. It is usually caused by calcification of a congenital bicuspid valve, age-related calcification of a normal aortic trileaflet valve, or rheumatic heart disease. Patients follow a well-defined disease course and rarely become symptomatic until older than 60 years. Once symptomatic with anginal symptoms, syncope, or congestive heart failure, patients have a precipitous decline in their clinical course and have an average survival of 2 to 5 years.[5]

Left-sided regurgitation
Acute left-sided regurgitation can be life threatening and patients often present in extremis. Acute aortic regurgitation is most often caused by infective endocarditis, aortic dissection, or blunt chest trauma. Acute mitral regurgitation is caused by flail leaflet or chordae tendinae rupture caused by infective endocarditis, blunt chest trauma, or myxomatous disease. It can also be caused by a papillary muscle rupture caused by ischemic disease. Regardless of aortic or mitral valve failure, the acute regurgitant volume leads to increased filling pressures and causes massive volume overload. Patients present with the sudden onset of pulmonary edema, hypotension, and cardiogenic shock.[6,7]

Infective endocarditis
A far less dramatic presentation, although also dangerous, can be seen with infective bacterial endocarditis, which may declare itself with little more than low-grade persistent fevers. The incidence and mortality of infective endocarditis has not decreased over the past 30 years. Although once a streptococcal disease affecting young adults with rheumatic heart disease, it is now predominantly a staphylococcal disease affecting a population with new risk factors. After staphylococci, viridans group streptococci and coagulase negative staphylococci are the most prevalent. Implanted prosthetic valves in an aging population are especially prone to become infected,

as are stenotic or incompetent native valves. Left-sided valves are more frequently infected. Right-sided endocarditis, particularly of the tricuspid valve, is particularly associated with intravenous (IV) drug abuse.[8,9]

Clinical Presentation and Work-up

Aortic stenosis

Patients with symptomatic aortic stenosis typically present with anginal symptoms, syncope, or congestive heart failure. It is imperative that emergency physicians carefully auscultate for a crescendo-decrescendo systolic ejection murmur in these patients, especially if given a history of aortic stenosis or having a loud murmur. Not being able to hear a harsh systolic murmur in these patients is a cause for alarm. It often signifies critical disease progression because the stenosed valve impedes forward blood flow causing the systolic ejection murmur to become more and more quiet. An ECG may show signs of left ventricular hypertrophy from the chronic disease process. A chest radiograph may show cardiomegaly and increased pulmonary congestion.[5] A poststenotic aortic dilatation is a characteristic finding.[10]

Left-sided regurgitation

Patients with an acute left-sided valvular regurgitation, whether from an incompetent aortic or mitral valve, present with an abrupt onset of symptoms, including dyspnea, pulmonary edema, hypotension, and cardiogenic shock. It is a challenging and time-sensitive diagnosis to make and requires a high degree of suspicion. Patients with an acute regurgitation are often tachycardic, tachypneic, and hypotensive with coarse rales and signs of heart failure on examination. Auscultation may yield a soft, early diastolic murmur. Patients with chronic, decompensated symptoms may have signs of left atrial enlargement or left ventricular hypertrophy on ECG or chest radiograph. Those with acute regurgitation will often have a normal ECG. A chest radiograph will show signs of mild pulmonary congestion in patients with chronic conditions and severe pulmonary edema in those with acute disease. All patients with suspected acute regurgitation should have an emergent echocardiogram.[11]

Infective endocarditis

Patients with acute infective endocarditis often present toxic in appearance with high fevers, chills, and rigors. Subacute infective endocarditis follows a more indolent course, and patients often have poorly localized symptoms with low-grade fevers, fatigue, and malaise. Infective endocarditis will rarely be definitively diagnosed in the ED because of the criteria needed for diagnosis. It must, however, always be suspected in patients with a fever, especially those with a new murmur or valvular risk factors. Fever is the most common vital sign abnormality. Acute phase reactants, such as C-reactive protein and erythrocyte sedimentation rate, are often elevated.[9]

The modified Duke criteria (**Table 1**) are the standard criteria used to guide the diagnosis of endocarditis.[12] The two major criteria are positive blood cultures and evidence of endocardial involvement on echocardiogram. There are also five minor criteria including fever, risk factors, and the classic signs of splinter hemorrhages, Janeway lesions and Roth spots—related to septic emboli to the fingernails, palms, and retina. The classic signs appear in a minority of patients, and their absence does not exclude the diagnosis of infective endocarditis. A firm diagnosis of endocarditis can be made by having either both major criteria, one major criteria and three minor criteria, or all five minor criteria. That sort of certainty, however, can be pursued on the in-patient services. In the Emergency Department, the goal is to entertain the diagnosis and begin the workup. Three sets of blood cultures should be drawn, with at least 1 hour apart between the first and third culture. At least one set should be

Table 1	
Modified Duke criteria for the diagnosis of infective endocarditis	
Major Criteria	Blood cultures positive for infective endocarditis
	Echocardiogram positive for infective endocarditis
Minor Criteria	Predisposition (predisposing heart condition or intravenous drug use)
	Fever greater than 38°C
	Vascular signs (ie, septic emboli, Janeway lesions)
	Immunologic signs (ie, Olser nodes, Roth spots)
	Microbiological evidence (ie, cultures, serology)

Adapted from Li JS, Sexton DJ, Mick N, et al. Modifications to the Duke criteria for the diagnosis of infective endocarditis. Clin Infect Dis 2000;30:633–8; with permission.

drawn from a separate site, given the possibility that patients may only intermittently shed bacteria to become bacteremic. Two sets of blood cultures have a sensitivity of approximately 95%, whereas 3 sets of blood cultures have a sensitivity of approximately 99%. Minor criteria include the classic signs of splinter hemorrhages, Janeway lesions, and Roth spots. These criteria are related to septic emboli to the fingernails, palms, and retina. They appear in a minority of patients, and the absence of these signs does not exclude the diagnosis of infective endocarditis.

Treatment and Management

Aortic stenosis
As previously noted, patients who are symptomatic with aortic stenosis, whether with angina, syncope, or congestive heart failure, have an average survival rate of 2 to 5 years from the onset of symptoms. Many cardiologists and cardiothoracic surgeons will consider valve replacement at the time of symptom onset. These patients should be admitted to the hospital for a formal echocardiogram to better evaluate the stenotic lesion and for the consideration of valve replacement.

In the ED, medical resuscitation of unstable patients with critical aortic stenosis involves aggressive fluid resuscitation because these patients are heavily preload dependent. Diuretics and nitrates to treat congestive heart failure should, thus, be used with caution in these patients to avoid a precipitous drop in systemic vascular resistance. There has been some recent evidence to suggest nitrates may be beneficial to promote contractility by alleviating left ventricular filling pressures and augmenting coronary blood flow. It should be noted that these patients were closely monitored with invasive devices in an intensive-care-unit (ICU) setting and nitrates should be used with caution in the ED.[13] When needed, inotropic medications, such as dopamine and dobutamine, are still more preferable than nitrates.

Surgical valve replacement is the definitive treatment. An intra-aortic balloon pump has been shown to be a useful adjunct in improving the hemodynamic stability of these patients while awaiting surgery.[14] Minimally invasive valve-replacement techniques are becoming increasingly common and are a promising treatment modality in the management of these patients who are often poor surgical candidates.[15]

Left-sided regurgitation
The management of acute left-sided regurgitation starts, as with all patients in the ED, with the ABCs: airway, breathing, and circulation. The airway often needs to be managed early in these patients, given the propensity to develop pulmonary edema from cardiogenic shock. Aggressive fluid resuscitation and inotropes to augment forward flow are the mainstays of medical therapy. Intra-aortic balloon pumps are

contraindicated for acute aortic regurgitation because they may augment the regurgitant volume through the aortic valve. They can be a useful adjunct for acute mitral regurgitation. Surgical valve replacement is the definitive treatment.[11]

Infective endocarditis

Emergency management of patients with suspected infective endocarditis includes drawing blood cultures, stabilizing patients hemodynamically, and starting the appropriate antibiotics. If patients are sent into the ED to rule out endocarditis with positive blood cultures from their outpatient provider, there are specific recommended antibiotic regimens. For undifferentiated patients with a suspicion of infective endocarditis, treatment depends on whether this infected valve is a native valve or prosthetic valve, and if a prosthetic valve, whether it is considered early (<12 months after surgery) or late.

Treatment of native valve endocarditis and late prosthetic valve endocarditis should cover infections caused by staphylococci, streptococci, HACEK (*Haemophilus, Actinobacillus, Cardiobacterium, Eikenella, Kingella*) species, and *Bartonella*. Proposed empiric antibiotic regimens include ampicillin-sulbactam or ampicillin-clavulanic acid with gentamicin; or vancomycin with gentamicin and ciprofloxacin. Treatment of early prosthetic valve endocarditis should include coverage of methicillin-resistant *Staphylococcus aureus*. The proposed empiric antibiotic regimen should include vancomycin with gentamicin and rifampin.[9]

ESSENTIAL QUESTIONS

How Should the Emergency Physician Approach the New, Asymptomatic Heart Murmur?

Some murmurs are incidental findings that, nevertheless, need an outpatient follow-up. The American College of Cardiologists (ACC) and the American Heart Association (AHA) recommend that no follow-up is needed if the murmur is midsystolic, grade II or softer, and thought to be innocent or functional by an experienced listener. But an asymptomatic murmur that is diastolic, continuous, holosystolic, late systolic, associated with ejection clicks, or that radiates to the neck or back needs to be evaluated by echocardiography.[16] There are no specific recommendations on the timing of this evaluation.

What are the Most Important Murmurs?

The answer to this question depends on the clinical context. In older patients who are febrile without an obvious source, any new murmur would be concerning because it could possibly indicate endocarditis. In a febrile IV drug user, a right-sided murmur is particularly telling, again as possibly indicating endocarditis, particularly of the tricuspid valve.

However, in reality there are probably only 3 major murmurs for which an ED physician requires expertise (**Table 2**). Two of them are the systolic murmurs of aortic stenosis and mitral regurgitation. Both of these murmurs occur with systole (ie,

Table 2	
Important valvular murmurs for the emergency practitioner	
Aortic stenosis	Systolic crescendo-decrescendo murmur heard best at the right upper sternal border with radiation to the carotids
Mitral regurgitation	Systolic murmur heard best over the cardiac apex with radiation to the axilla
Aortic regurgitation	Diastolic murmur heard best at the left sternal borders

immediately after or instead of the S1 heart sound). Aortic stenosis is generally heard loudest at the right upper sternal border and radiates to the carotids. Mitral regurgitation is generally heard over the apex of the heart and radiates to the axilla. A third important valvular problem, aortic regurgitation, presents with a blowing diastolic murmur (ie, a soft murmur immediately after or instead of the S2 heart sound). In patients with ripping or tearing back pain, such a soft-blowing murmur after S2 could herald a life-threatening aortic dissection or aneurysm.

How can the Emergency Physician Determine What Kind of Prosthetic Valve Patients have?

It is useful to identify the type of prosthetic valve that patients have implanted, especially to guide auscultation for abnormal heart sounds. When the ED physician does not hear the expected sounds on auscultation, he or she must be acutely concerned for valve malfunction. Some rules of thumb include the following: Prosthetic aortic valves should produce a closing click at the end of systole (during S2). Prosthetic mitral valves should produce a late diastolic click (closing as S1 begins). Tissue valve closing sounds mimic native valves, and you may hear a normal S1 and S2 with no murmur.

Patients are instructed to carry cards in their wallets identifying the serial number and the type of valve that they have implanted along with the surgeon and the hospital at which the operation took place. If this information is not available, chest radiography is of immense value in identifying the type of mechanical valve.

The lateral radiograph is the most useful. Bisecting the heart in half and also from the apex to the base divides the lateral chest radiograph into 4 regions: The aortic valve is in the anterosuperior region. The pulmonic valve is in the posterosuperior region. The tricuspid valve is in the anteroinferior region. The mitral valve is in the posteroinferior region. Anteroposterior radiography can be similarly used, but it is less reliable because the valves are closer in proximity to one another. Dividing the heart into 4 regions again: The aortic valve is in the left upper quadrant. The pulmonic valve is in the right upper quadrant. The mitral valve is in the left lower quadrant. The mitral valve is in the right lower quadrant. Chest radiography is also useful in identifying the direction the valve is pointing. For example, the direction of a valve along the aortic outflow tract may suggest that it is an aortic valve.

When is Prophylactic Antibiotic Therapy Mandated in Patients with Prosthetic Valves?

The percentage of valves that become infected is 1% to 6%, an incidence rate that has prompted the practice of giving antibiotics prophylactically to patients with artificial heart valves, congenital heart disease, or a history of endocarditis.[17]

The AHA and the ACC recently updated their 2008 guidelines regarding such prophylaxis. The AHA/ACC guidelines now recommend a single dose of antibiotic (typically, amoxicillin 2 g by mouth) given 30 to 60 minutes before dental procedures that manipulate the gingival tissue or the periapical region or perforate the oral mucosa. In patients allergic to penicillins, the guidelines recommend a cephalosporin or macrolide (cephalexin 2 g or azithromycin 500 mg, for example). Patients who cannot take oral antibiotics can be given ampicillin, cefazolin, clindamycin, or ceftriaxone doses intravenously.[18]

Routine prophylactic antibiotics are no longer indicated for wound management or for gastrointestinal, genitourinary, or respiratory tract procedures. So, it is safe to perform a bronchoscopy or a transesophageal echo, place a Foley catheter, incise and drain an abscess, or suture up a minor laceration without prior antibiotics. The

AHA/ACC guideline committee does note that some clinicians may wish to continue antibiotic prophylaxis for patients with bicuspid aortic valve, coarctation of the aorta, severe mitral valve prolapse, or hypertrophic obstructive cardiomyopathy.[18]

What are the Early Complications Associated with a Recently Implanted Artificial Heart Valve?

Prosthetic heart valve complications can be divided into early (within 3 months of surgery) and late complications (>3 months from surgery). The most dangerous complication in the early postoperative period is pericardial effusion leading to cardiac tamponade. Cardiac tamponade occurs when fluid accumulates in the pericardium causing compression of the right ventricle during diastole. This condition leads to the bowing of the ventricular septum into the left ventricle causing decreased stroke volume and signs of obstructive shock. Patients classically present with Beck triad of hypotension, jugular venous distension, and muffled heart sounds. A measured pulsus paradoxus of greater than 10 mmHg is suggestive of tamponade physiology.[19,20]

Bedside ultrasonography by the emergency practitioner can expeditiously diagnose cardiac tamponade before formal echocardiography. Classic echocardiographic signs of tamponade include visualizing right ventricular diastolic collapse and also seeing cardiac alternans, the swinging of the heart within the pericardial effusion. One can also see the pathophysiology behind pulsus paradoxus as previously described and visualize right ventricular dilation with inspiration and compression with expiration. It is also useful to visualize the inferior vena cava (IVC) using M mode under sonography. The increased right atrial filling pressures cause persistent IVC dilation with minimal (if any) respiratory variation.[21]

The emergency treatment is pericardiocentesis. Postoperative patients, however, are likely to have clotted blood in the pericardial sac that may be difficult to aspirate with a needle. If needle pericardiocentesis is unsuccessful, the patients' freshly closed midline sternotomy incision can be opened with a scalpel and a gloved hand can be inserted into the pericardium to remove the clot.[22]

Atrial fibrillation is another complication that often occurs after the operation. It should be managed with antiarrhythmics in conjunction with the patients' cardiothoracic surgeon.[20]

A postoperative inflammation of the pericardium can also be seen and is termed postpericardiotomy syndrome. It usually presents 1 to 6 weeks after an operation and patients typically present with fever, pleuritic chest pain, pain worse in the supine position, or shortness of breath. Pleural effusions or cardiomegaly (secondary to associated pericardial effusion) may be seen on chest radiograph. ECG may show diffuse ST elevation and PR depression as this is an inflammatory condition similar to pericarditis. Laboratory values may be remarkable for leukocytosis, elevated sedimentation rate, and elevated C-reactive protein. Treatment is with antiinflammatory medications or corticosteroids.[20]

What are the Late Complications Associated with a Long-Standing Artificial Heart Valve?

Late complications associated with an implanted artificial heart valve relate largely with anticoagulation. Patients that are inadequately anticoagulated may present with heart valve thrombosis. Patients with an acute thrombosis of a heart valve present with signs and symptoms of obstructive shock. The diagnosis is made by echocardiography. The treatment of unstable patients is thrombolysis followed by anticoagulation. Patients unresponsive to thrombolysis must be taken emergently to the operating room.[23]

Mechanical valves can fracture and prosthetic valves can be worn down. Patients with a leaflet fracture or ruptured valve present in extremis with acute onset shortness of breath, pulmonary edema, and shock. In the ED, these patients need to be emergently intubated and receive fluids, pressors, and inotropes while awaiting definitive surgical management. They should also get an emergent echocardiogram, either in the ED or the ICU.[24]

When can Anticoagulation be Reversed in Patients with an Artificial Heart Valve?

By creating turbulent blood flow and shearing forces, artificial heart valves create a predisposition to form clots (which, as in atrial fibrillation, can then be showered off through the arterial system as emboli). Patients with mechanical valves, thus, need to be on lifelong anticoagulation, with relatively high target international normalized ratios (INRs). The usual range is from 2.5 to 3.5. Only the ball-and-cage model of aortic valve has a lower INR target of 2.0 to 3.0. Bioprosthetic valves, such as porcine valve transplants, are less thrombogenic and, thus, generally only require anticoagulation for the first 3 months.[25]

Given the high risk for thrombosis, and the correspondingly aggressive anticoagulation, it is not surprising that a major concern with patients with artificial heart valves revolves around the risk for clotting or bleeding events.

Emergent reversal of anticoagulation, in the face of life-threatening gastrointestinal bleeding, trauma, or hemorrhagic stroke, for example, can be accomplished with fresh frozen plasma (FFP). The use of FFP is preferable to the use of vitamin K for fear of creating a hypercoagulable state with high-dose vitamin K and to enable more precise control over lowering the INR to a target level.[16]

There is a paucity of data on the safety of reversing anticoagulation. Anecdotally, there have been cases of thromboembolism of a valve from a subtherapeutic INR in just 1 to 2 days. For example, one of the authors managed a patient with a subarachnoid hemorrhage and a St. Jude valve whose anticoagulation was reversed for just 24 hours. Within 2 hours of reinitiating anticoagulation with a heparin bridge, the patient developed left-sided facial and arm paralysis, initially raising concern that her hemorrhage was expanding. Her heparin was turned off while emergent head imaging was arranged; this revealed not an expansion of the bleeding, but a new ischemic stroke, likely from the artificial valve.

One retrospective study looked at 28 patients with mechanical valves that needed anticoagulation in the setting of a life-threatening bleed. The patients received vitamin K or FFP, and anticoagulation was withheld for 11 to 19 days. The study noted that none of the patients had thromboembolic complications from their valves, although there were 4 in-hospital deaths from bleeding complications. The conclusion was that the thromboembolic risk is low in patients with prosthetic valves hospitalized for life-threatening bleed when anticoagulation is held.[26]

How Safely can Anticoagulation be Held in Patients with an Artificial Heart Valve?

There may be circumstances when an emergency practitioner is involved in coordinating an elective procedure for a patient and may be asked to withhold anticoagulation. According to the ACC/AHA guidelines, patients with a modern, bileaflet mechanical aortic valve and no other risk factors are at a relatively low risk for valve-related thrombosis. In fact, when these patients are headed for an elective procedure of some sort, the recommended approach is to simply hold warfarin therapy for 2 to 3 days, enough so that INR decreases less than 1.5, and then restart warfarin a day after the procedure, with no heparin bridging.[16]

The risk of a valve-related thrombosis is much higher for artificial mitral or tricuspid valves. Patients are also considered high risk for thrombosis if they have any mechanical valve associated with additional risk factors, including atrial fibrillation, left ventricular dysfunction, a previous thromboembolism, or a known hypercoagulable condition. For these high-risk patients, warfarin is also held before elective surgery or procedures. But therapeutic heparin dosing is added in when the INR decreases to less than 2 (typically 48 hours before surgery), with heparin stopped only 4 to 6 hours before the procedure and reinitiated as soon afterwards as bleeding stability allows.[16]

REFERENCES

1. Zipes D, Libby P, Bonow R. Braunwald's Heart Disease: a textbook of cardiovascular medicine, vol. 66. 9th edition. Philadelphia: Elsevier Saunders; 2012. p. 1468.
2. Vongpatanasin W, Hillis LD, Lange RA. Prosthetic heart valves. N Engl J Med 1996;335:407–16.
3. Nishimura RA, Carabello BA, Faxon DP, et al. ACC/AHA guidelines for the management of patients with valvular heart disease. J Am Coll Cardiol 1998; 32:486–588.
4. Bruce CJ, Connolly HM. Right-sided valve disease deserves a little more respect. Circulation 2009;119:2726–34.
5. Carabello BA, Paulus WJ. Aortic stenosis. The Lancet 2009;373:956–66.
6. Bekeredjian R, Grayburn PA. Aortic regurgitation. Circulation 2005;112:125–34.
7. Enriquez-Sarano M, Akins CW, Vahanian A. Mitral regurgitation. The Lancet 2009; 373:1382–94.
8. de Sa DD, Tleyjeh IM, Anavekar NS, et al. Epidemiological trends of infective endocarditis: a population-based study in Olmsted County, Minnesota. Mayo Clin Proc 2010;85:422–6.
9. Habib G, Hoen B, Tornos P, et al. Guidelines on the prevention, diagnosis, and treatment of infective endocarditis. Eur Heart J 2009;30:2369–413.
10. Wilton E, Jahangiri M. Post-stenotic aortic dilatation. J Cardiothorac Surg 2006; 1:7.
11. Mokadam NA, Stout KK, Verrier ED. Management of acute regurgitation in left-sided cardiac valves. Tex Heart Inst J 2011;38:9–19.
12. Li JS, Sexton DJ, Mick N, et al. Modifications to the Duke criteria for the diagnosis of infective endocarditis. Clin Infect Dis 2000;30:633–8.
13. Khot UN, Novaro GM, Popović ZB, et al. Nitroprusside in critically ill patients with left ventricular dysfunction and aortic stenosis. N Engl J Med 2003;348:1756–63.
14. Aksoy O, Yousefzai R, Singh D, et al. Cardiogenic shock in the setting of severe aortic stenosis: role of intra-aortic balloon pump support. Heart 2011;97(10): 838–43.
15. Leon MB, Smith CR, Mack M, et al. Transcatheter aortic-valve implantation for aortic stenosis in patients who cannot undergo surgery. N Engl J Med 2010; 363:1597–607.
16. Bonow RO, Carabello BA, Chatterjee K. 2008 focused update incorporated into the ACC/AHA 2006 guidelines for the management of patients with valvular heart disease. Circulation 2008;118:e523–661.
17. Mandell GL, Bennett JE, Dolin R. Mandell, Douglas, and Bennett's principles and practice of infectious diseases. 7th edition. Philadelphia: Churchill Livingstone Elsevier 2010;78:1113.

18. Nishimura RA, Carabello BA, Freed MD, et al. ACC/AHA 2008 guideline update on valvular heart disease: focused update on infective endocarditis. Circulation 2008;118:887–96.
19. Spodick DH. Acute cardiac tamponade. N Engl J Med 2003;349:684–90.
20. Maisch B, Seferović PM, Ristić AD, et al. Guidelines on the diagnosis and management of pericardial diseases executive summary. Eur Heart J 2004;25: 587–610.
21. Echocardiography in the ICU: Tamponade. Available at: https://www.stanford.edu/group/ccm_echocardio/cgi-bin/mediawiki/index.php/Tamponade. Accessed June 1, 2011.
22. Whittle JS, Parrish GA, Rosenberg MS, et al. Complications of prosthetic heart valves in the emergency department. Emerg Med Rep 2010;31:41.
23. Larsen GL, Alexander JA, Stanford W. Thromboembolic phenomena in patients with prosthetic aortic valves who did not receive anticoagulants. Ann Thorac Surg 1977;23:323–6.
24. Lengyel M, Fuster V, Keltai M, et al. Guidelines for management of left-sided prosthetic valve thrombosis: a role for thrombolytic therapy. J Am Coll Cardiol 1977; 30:1521–6.
25. Bloomfield P. Choice of heart valve prosthesis. Heart 2002;87:583–609.
26. Ananthasubramaniam K, Beattie JN, Rosman HS, et al. How safely and for how long can warfarin therapy be withheld in prosthetic heart valve patients hospitalized with a major hemorrhage? Chest 2001;119:478–84.

Congenital Heart Disease

Katherine Dolbec, MD[a],*, Nathan W. Mick, MD[b]

KEYWORDS

- Pediatric • Congenital heart disease
- Echocardiography • Cardiology

Congenital heart disease is estimated to affect up to 1% of live births, although the spectrum of disease severity varies greatly.[1] Severe lesions, such as hypoplastic left heart syndrome or truncus arteriosus, are relatively rare compared with atrial or ventricular septal defects and some lesions, such as a small patent ductus arteriosus, may resolve spontaneously.[2] Despite advances in diagnosis and surgical care, congenital cardiac malformations remain one of the leading cause of death in infants.[3] The incidence of specific congenital heart disease lesions is reflected in **Table 1**. Most congenital heart disease is diagnosed in utero by ultrasound during routine prenatal care. However, some lesions may escape detection and not manifest until after birth (**Table 2**), and these are the ones that are most likely to present to the emergency department. A significant proportion of lesions is dependent on mixing of oxygenated and deoxygenated blood and relies on a patent ductus arteriosus for communication between the systemic and pulmonic circulations. Thus, a child with congenital heart disease may present with severe cyanosis or shock at 1 to 2 weeks of age as the ductus arteriosus closes, making an understanding of these lesions crucial for any clinician who treats children in the neonatal period. Some nonobstructive lesions (ie, ventricular septal defects and patent ductus arteriosus) present later in the newborn period with congestive heart failure (CHF). The cardinal presentations of cyanosis, shock, and CHF can mimic those of pulmonary disease or sepsis; thus, the emergency physician must establish a broad differential and consider congenital heart disease when treating a critically ill neonate. Along with structural abnormalities, congenital rhythm disturbances, such as supraventricular tachycardia, congenital complete heart block, and long QTc syndrome, can also present during the newborn period with signs and symptoms that suggest other, more common conditions.

The authors have nothing to disclose.
[a] Department of Emergency Medicine, Maine Medical Center, 22 Bramhall Street, Portland, ME 04102, USA
[b] Pediatric Emergency Medicine, Department of Emergency Medicine, Maine Medical Center, 22 Bramhall Street, Portland, ME 04102, USA
* Corresponding author.
E-mail address: dolbek@mmc.org

Emerg Med Clin N Am 29 (2011) 811–827
doi:10.1016/j.emc.2011.08.005
0733-8627/11/$ – see front matter © 2011 Elsevier Inc. All rights reserved.

Table 1
Incidence of specific congenital heart defects

Lesion	Estimated Percentage of Congenital Heart Disease
Ventricular septal defect	20%
Tetralogy of Fallot	10%
Atrial septal defect	5%
Tricuspid atresia	1%
Pulmonary stenosis	1%
Transposition of the great vessels	5%
Ebstein anomaly	1%
Coarctation of the aorta	10%
Critical aortic stenosis	5%
Interrupted aortic arch	1%
Hypoplastic left heart syndrome	1%
Patent ductus arteriosus	10%

ANATOMY AND PATHOPHYSIOLOGY

Circulation in the fetus is designed to transport oxygen-rich blood from the placenta to the systemic circulation. To accomplish this feat, the fetal lungs must be bypassed and blood shunted from the right side of the heart to the left. After leaving the placenta, oxygen-rich blood bypasses the liver through the ductus venosus and is returned to the right atrium. Most of this oxygenated blood then travels from the right atrium to the left atrium through the foramen ovale and is then pumped to the systemic circulation by the left ventricle. A small amount of blood enters the high-resistance pulmonary circuit and then is shunted right to left across the ductus arteriousus, from the pulmonary artery to the aortic arch.

At birth, the lungs fill with air, and the pulmonary vascular resistance drops dramatically. This leads to a complex series of changes that results in the normal circulatory pattern seen in adults. As the pulmonary vascular resistance falls, more blood enters

Table 2
Time of presentation of specific congenital heart defects

Lesion	Time of Presentation
Ventricular septal defect	After 4 weeks
Tetralogy of Fallot	Birth to 12 weeks
Tricuspid atresia	Birth to 2 weeks
Pulmonary stenosis/atresia	Birth to 2 weeks
Transposition of the great vessels	Birth to 2 weeks
Ebstein anomaly	Birth to 2 weeks
Coarctation of the aorta	1–2 weeks for critical lesions, later if less severe
Aortic stenosis	1–2 weeks for critical lesions, later if less severe
Interrupted aortic arch	Birth to 2 weeks
Hypoplastic left heart syndrome	Birth to 2 weeks
Patent ductus arteriosus	After 4 weeks

the pulmonary circuit and oxygenated blood is delivered in larger quantities to the left atrium. This leads to a reversal of pressure forces and functional closure of the foramen ovale. During this time of transition, systemic vascular resistance rises and results in a reversal of shunting through the ductus. The blood flowing left to right across the ductus arteriosus is now highly oxygenated and this results in closure of this pathway within the first 2 weeks of life. The increased workload on the left ventricle results in an increased left ventricular mass while the right ventricle mass decreases. Normal fetal circulatory anatomy is depicted in **Fig. 1**. The development of the heart is a complex embryologic process involving an organized series of molecular and morphogenetic events. Any genetic, molecular, or cellular error in this process can result in gross structural abnormalities of the heart, heart valves, blood vessels, or conduction system with functional significance.[4] There are many risk factors for the development of congenital heart disease. Family history plays a role; 1% to 4% of babies born to parents with congenital heart disease are affected.[5] Maternal diabetes is associated with up to a 30% chance of structural heart disease in the newborn, particularly hypertrophic cardiomyopathy, ventricular septal defect, or transposition of the great vessels (TOGV).[6] Maternal alcohol or drug use (ie, lithium use and associated Ebstein anomaly) also increases the risk of heart defects (**Table 3**).

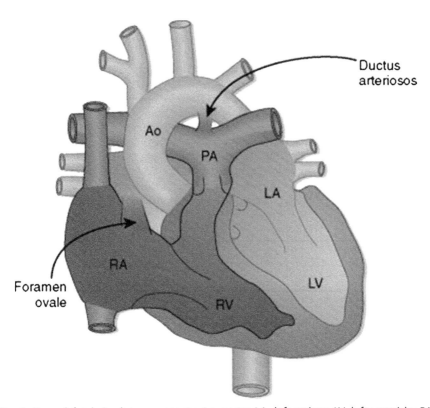

Fig. 1. Normal fetal circulatory anatomy. Ao, aorta; LA, left atrium; LV, left ventricle; PA, pulmonary artery; RA, right atrium; RV, right ventricle. (*From* Mick N. Pediatric cardiac disorders. In: Adams JG, Barton ED, Collings J, et al, editors. Emergency medicine. 1st edition. Philadelphia: Saunders Elsevier; 2008. p. 618; with permission.)

Table 3	
Congenital heart disease risk factors	
Risk Factor	**Lesions Associated**
Maternal diabetes	Ventricular septal defect, transposition of the great vessels, hypertrophic cardiomyopathy
Maternal lithium use	Ebstein anomaly
Maternal phenytoin use	Aortic stenosis, pulmonic stenosis
Maternal alcohol use	Ventricular septal defect, atrial septal defect

DIAGNOSIS AND STABILIZATION OF SUSPECTED CONGENITAL HEART DISEASE

Neonates presenting to the emergency department with undiagnosed congenital heart disease, whether it be structural or arrhythmogenic, typically exhibit signs of shock, cyanosis, CHF, or a combination of the three and typically present at 2 weeks of age as the ductus arteriosus closes. Those with left-sided obstructive lesions present with inadequate systemic perfusion and shock, whereas those with right-sided lesions present with cyanosis because of inadequate blood reaching the lungs. The differential diagnosis of shock in a neonate is broad with infectious etiologies being far and away the most common (**Table 4**). A blood pressure differential between the preductal right arm and the postductal left arm may suggest a ductal-dependent left-sided obstructive lesion, such as critical coarctation of the aorta or congenital aortic stenosis.

Cyanosis is caused by the presence of deoxygenated blood at the level of the capillaries. Detection of cyanosis requires a systemic oxygen saturation of 80% to 85%, depending on the patient's hemoglobin level. Transient peripheral cyanosis (acrocyanosis) can occur in children with normal cardiac anatomy and function as a result of benign conditions, such as cold exposure, and more serious noncardiac conditions, such as sepsis. Central cyanosis, involving the mucous membranes, the lips, or the trunk, is always pathologic and should raise red flags. In children with cyanotic congenital heart disease, cyanosis can occur if blood flow to the lungs is insufficient or if a large percentage of the deoxygenated blood is pumped to the systemic circulation and a large percentage of the oxygenated blood is pumped back to the lungs.[7]

Table 4	
Differential diagnosis of shock in the neonate	
Type of Shock	**Etiology**
Hypovolemia	Dehydration
	Blood loss
Cardiogenic	Coarctation of the aorta
	Aortic stenosis
	Interrupted aortic arch
	Hypoplastic left heart syndrome
	Congenital arrythmias
	Myocarditis
	Tension pneumothorax
	Tamponade
Distributive	Sepsis
	Anaphylaxis

Pulmonary causes of cyanosis typically improve with supplemental oxygen administration or agitation, whereas cardiac cyanosis does not improve with oxygen and generally worsens with activity or crying.[8] Neonates who present with cyanosis generally have ductal-dependent right-sided obstructive lesions and are intolerant of the transition to postnatal circulation.

CHF occurs with structural heart disease and congenital rhythm abnormalities. Typically, the infant presents with respiratory distress, tachypnea, and rales on pulmonary examination, although more subtle signs, such as poor feeding and sweating with feeds, may be the only clue to the diagnosis. Unlike adults with CHF, peripheral edema is rare in children. Physical examination findings suggestive of heart failure include signs of respiratory distress with grunting, flaring, and pulmonary rales. Hepatomegaly is also a common sign caused by engorgement of the hepatic vasculature, and examination of the liver edge should be a standard part of the examination in any child presenting in the first month of life with respiratory distress. Heart failure can be caused by volume overload of the right ventricle as is seen in total anomalous pulmonary venous return (TAPVR) with a large ventricular septal defect or lesions with large left-to-right shunts, such as critical aortic stenosis or coarctation of the aorta as blood preferentially flows into the low resistance pulmonary circuit. Congenital rhythm disturbances, particularly supraventricular tachycardia, can also lead to CHF because of poor cardiac output. For the emergency physician, initial management should be focused on the stabilization of these cardinal presentations.

STABILIZING DUCTAL-DEPENDENT LEFT-SIDED OBSTRUCTIVE LESIONS PRESENTING AS SHOCK

Ductal-dependent left-sided obstructive lesions include coarctation of the aorta, critical aortic stenosis, interrupted aortic arch, and hypoplastic left heart syndrome. These lesions are similar in that blood flow to the systemic circulation is contingent on the patency of the ductus arteriosus (**Fig. 2**). Many of these lesions are detected in utero by the 20-week anatomic ultrasound during the prenatal period. If undetected, they become apparent during the first 2 weeks of life when the ductus arteriosus closes and these infants typically present with profound shock and without cyanosis. The differential diagnosis of shock in the neonate is broad and includes cardiac, infectious, and metabolic causes. All neonates in shock should be treated aggressively with intubation if necessary; fluid resuscitation (20 mL/kg of normal saline); and empiric antibiotics and antivirals (ampicillin, gentamicin, and acyclovir). If the infant fails to

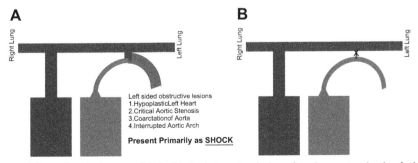

Fig. 2. (A) Preductal closure of left-sided obstructive lesion showing systemic circulation dependent on patent ductus arteriosus and mixing occurring at the level of the ductus. (B) Closure of the ductus results in decrease in systemic perfusion and shock.

respond to these interventions or a cardiac cause is suspected, prostaglandin E_1 should be given. Prostaglandin E_1 is given as an infusion starting at 0.1 μg/kg/min and works by preventing closure of the ductus arteriosus, which results in improved systemic blood flow in left-sided obstructive lesions. The infusion is titrated to palpable femoral pulses and positive results occur in minutes. The major side effect of the infusion is apnea, which can occur in up to 10% of patients and intubation should be considered if an infant is to be transferred to another facility.[9] Once a child has been stabilized on prostaglandins, definitive management involves consultation with a pediatric cardiologist for echocardiography and transfer to a center capable of repairing the lesion in question.

STABILIZING DUCTAL-DEPENDENT RIGHT-SIDED OBSTRUCTIVE LESIONS PRESENTING AS CYANOSIS

Ductal-dependent right-sided obstructive lesions include tricuspid atresia, severe pulmonic stenosis, tetralogy of Fallot, TOGV, Ebstein anomaly, and many others. In right-sided obstruction, pulmonary blood flow is dependent on the combined volume of that coming from the ductus arteriosis and that coming through the obstructed right ventricular output. As the ductus closes, at 1 to 2 weeks of age, the infant becomes cyanotic (**Fig. 3**). The differential diagnosis of cyanosis includes cardiac and pulmonary conditions, and chest radiographs and the hyperoxia test may be useful in making the distinction. A chest radiograph is obtained looking for signs of pulmonary disease including pneumothorax, lung collapse, or pneumonia, and to evaluate the heart size and shape. The hyperoxia test takes advantage of the fact that supplemental oxygen does not raise the Pao_2 of the blood in congenital heart disease to the same degree as in pulmonary disease because of the presence of an intracardiac shunt. To perform the test, have the infant breath 100% oxygen for 10 minutes and then measure a postductal arterial blood gas. Congenital heart disease is suggested if the Pao_2 is less than 150 mm Hg during hyperoxia. Pulmonary disease is more likely if the Pao_2 is greater than 150 mm Hg during hyperoxia.

Stabilizing right-sided obstructive lesions involves the administration of a prostaglandin E_1 infusion to keep the ductus arteriosus open. The dosing of prostaglandins is identical to that used in left-sided obstruction and the infusion should be titrated to oxygen saturations of 80% to 85%. Once the oxygen saturations have been stabilized,

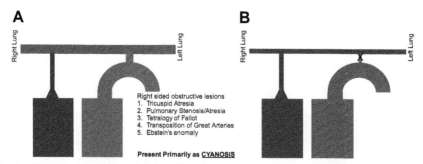

Fig. 3. (*A*) Preductal closure of right-sided obstructive lesion showing pulmonary circulation dependent on patent ductus arteriosus and mixing occurring at the level of the ductus. (*B*) Closure of the ductus results in severe cyanosis because oxygenated blood from the lungs has no way to enter the systemic circuit.

pediatric cardiology consultation should be obtained and transfer to an appropriate tertiary care center effected.

STABILIZATION OF LESIONS PRESENTING WITH CHF

Treatment of CHF in the newborn suspected of having congenital heart disease may require intubation and positive pressure ventilation, and gentle diuresis. Because structural heart disease and congenital rhythm abnormalities can cause CHF, electrocardiography early in the resuscitation may aid in the diagnosis. Supraventricular tachycardia in infants is suggested by a narrow complex tachycardia with rates greater than 220 beats per minute.

LESION-SPECIFIC PRESENTATIONS
Left-sided Obstructive Lesions

Hypoplastic left heart syndrome
Hypoplastic left heart syndrome is a spectrum of cardiac anomalies including varying degrees of underdevelopment of the aorta, aortic valve, left ventricle, mitral valve, and left atrium. The right ventricle is the dominant pumping chamber of the heart and systemic blood flow relies on right-to-left shunting via the ductus arteriosus to the aorta.

Before closure of the ductus arteriosus, patients may have subtle signs including mild cyanosis, tachypnea, and tachycardia. When the ductus arteriosus begins to constrict, systemic cardiac output is significantly reduced and profound CHF, cardiovascular collapse, and shock rapidly develops.

Chest radiographs may reveal cardiomegaly with pulmonary edema. Electrocardiogram is generally nonspecific but may show evidence of right ventricular hypertrophy. Definitive diagnosis requires echocardiography, which can elucidate the character and severity of the anatomic anomalies. Initial stabilization involves prostaglandin E_1 infusion and endotracheal intubation is frequently required.[10]

Coarctation of the aorta
Coarctation of the aorta represents a spectrum of disease ranging from mild narrowing of the descending aorta to complete interruption of the aortic arch. It most often presents as a discrete narrowing in the region of the ligamentum arteriosum. The descending aorta just proximal to the coarcted section is frequently aneurismal, and a bicuspid aortic valve is present in between 22% and 42% of cases.[11] After closure of the ductus arteriosus, infants with severe coarctation or an interrupted aortic arch present in shock with acidosis and evidence of end-organ damage.

The most significant clue to diagnosis is a pulse differential between the upper and lower extremities. A normal patient has an increase of 5 to 10 mm in systolic blood pressure in the lower extremities compared with the upper extremities. Absence of this differential or a decrease in the systolic blood pressure in the lower extremities compared with the upper extremities should prompt further evaluation for coarctation. Chest radiograph may demonstrate characteristic rib notching, indicative of significant arterial collateral formation bypassing the coarcted area. Echocardiography is again the diagnostic modality of choice and initial stabilization involves prostaglandin E_1 infusion, inotropic support with dopamine or dobutamine, and correction of acidosis with bicarbonate.

Aortic stenosis
Aortic stenosis is defined as narrowing across the aortic valve. Left untreated, this results in increased afterload on the left ventricle, left ventricular hypertrophy, and

eventual dilatation and failure of the left ventricle. In neonates with critical aortic valvular stenosis, shock caused by an obstructed aortic valve puts these infants at extreme risk for early sudden death.[3]

Echocardiography is used to confirm the diagnosis and prostaglandin E_1 is a life-saving intervention in patients with critical aortic stenosis. Initial stabilization also includes airway support, inotropic augmentation with dopamine or dobutamine, and correction of acidosis.[8]

Right-sided Obstructive Lesions

Transposition of the great vessels

TOGV accounts for 5% of congenital heart disease in children.[4] Half of the patients with this anomaly present within the first hour of life and 90% present within the first day.[12] With this lesion, the aorta arises from the right ventricle and receives deoxygenated blood returning from the systematic circulation. This results in oxygen saturations in the main pulmonary artery that exceed those in the aorta. Infants with transposition of the great arteries may be at higher risk of cerebral damage than others because of chronically decreased oxygen delivery to the brain in fetal life as oxygenated blood is pumped preferentially to the lower body at the expense of the brain.[13] With the two components of the circulation working in parallel instead of in series, a connection between the two, at the level of the atria, the ventricles, or the ductus, is required for survival.

Neonates with TOGV develop cyanosis soon after birth as the mixing between venous and arterial blood diminishes with the closure of the foramen ovale and the ductus arteriosus. If an atrial septal defect, ventricular septal defect, or patent ductus arteriosus is present, mixing is improved, and cyanosis may not present immediately. Respirations are typically not labored, the liver is not enlarged, and pulses are generally normal. There is usually not a murmur.

Chest radiographs in TOGV typically show a normal or minimally enlarged cardiac silhouette. The superior mediastinum is usually narrow and the thymus is involuted, which leads to an "egg-on-a-string" appearance (**Fig. 4**). Pulmonary vasculature is prominent, and the aortic arch is left-sided. A normal chest radiograph does not exclude the diagnosis of transposition, and the classic findings are seen less than 50% of the time.[14]

Echocardiography is the test of choice for diagnosing TOGV and can also be helpful in identifying associated lesions, such as pulmonic valvular stenosis, a patent foramen ovale, and ventricular and atrial septal defects. Significant aortic arch hypoplasia, interruption, or coarctation occurs in 19% of infants with TOGV and an associated ventricular septal defect and in 0.6% of patients with an intact ventricular septum.[13] Echocardiography can also help the clinician visualize the response of the patent ductus arteriosus to a prostaglandin infusion.

Tetralogy of Fallot

Tetralogy of Fallot is the most common cyanotic congenital heart defect. Hallmarks of this lesion are (1) large, nonrestrictive ventricular septal defect; (2) severe right ventricular outflow track obstruction; (3) overriding of the aorta; and (4) right ventricular hypertrophy. Timing of presentation and degree of cyanosis correlates precisely with the amount of right ventricular outflow tract obstruction. Patients with severe outflow tract obstruction (blue tets) present early in the neonatal period. Those patients with adequate pulmonary blood flow at birth (pink tets) gradually develop increasing cyanosis during the first few weeks and months of life. These patients may present to the emergency department with hypercyanotic "tet" spells, which occur as a consequence of transient reductions in pulmonary blood flow.[15]

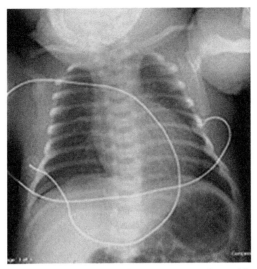

Fig. 4. Egg-on-a-string appearance of the mediastinum in a patient with transposition of the great vessels. (*From* Geggel R, editor. Multimedia library of congenital heart disease. Boston: Children's Hospital; Available at: www.childrenshospital.org/mml/cvp. Accessed April 19, 2007; with permission.)

Cyanosis is the most common presenting complaint in infants with tetralogy who are not diagnosed in utero. Hypercyanotic tet spells are the most dramatic presentation of this condition and are characterized by profound cyanosis, respiratory distress and grunting, and fussiness and agitation. These spells are brought on by increased right-to-left shunting and should be treated in a stepwise fashion with oxygen, knee-chest position, morphine sulfate, β-blockade, and phenylephrine.[16] Knee-chest positioning of the infant is thought to increase systemic vascular resistance and decrease right-to-left shunting. Morphine acts to calm agitation and decrease venous return. β-Blockade slows the heart rate and allows more blood to enter the pulmonary circuit across the right ventricular outflow tract, and phenylephrine infusion increases systemic vascular resistance. Tetralogy of Fallot may also be suggested on chest radiography by the presence of a "boot-shaped" heart, which is caused by the absence of the small, atretic pulmonary arteries (**Fig. 5**), although diagnosis is most often made by echocardiography.[17]

Ebstein anomaly

Ebstein anomaly is a cardiac abnormality of the tricuspid valve and right ventricle in which the valve is displaced downward and there is "atrialization" of a portion of the ventricle.[18] This lesion is associated with tricuspid valvular insufficiency and stenosis, and patients with these anomalies often have accessory atrioventricular conduction pathways or intraventricular conduction delays that predispose them to arrhythmias. Patients can also have other structural cardiac anomalies, the most common of which is an atrial septal defect, which occurs in 80% to 94% of patients with Ebstein anomaly.[19] Patients presenting with Ebstein anomaly have a high mortality rate, with one study showing that 18% of newborns presenting with Ebstein anomaly died in the neonatal period.[20]

Ebstein anomaly may present with cyanosis, right-sided heart failure, arrhythmias, or sudden cardiac death. Prognosis in these patients is determined by degree of cyanosis and presence or absence of arrhythmias.

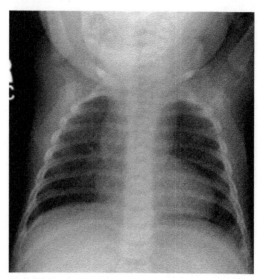

Fig. 5. The boot-shaped heart characteristic of tetralogy of Fallot. (*From* Geggel R, editor. Multimedia library of congenital heart disease. Boston: Children's Hospital; Available at: www.childrenshospital.org/mml/cvp. Accessed April 19, 2007; with permission.)

Chest radiographs reveal dramatic cardiomegaly, sometimes so extreme that the heart occupies most of the thoracic cavity. The heart is described as "globe-shaped" and may have a narrow waist. Echocardiography is the test of choice for diagnosing Ebstein anomaly and demonstrates the degree of inferior displacement of the proximal attachments of the tricuspid valvular septal leaflet.

An electrocardiogram should be obtained, because patients with Ebstein anomaly often have associated arrhythmias.[20] Other electrocardiographic abnormalities seen with Ebstein anomaly include tall and broad P waves, prolonged PR interval, and complete or incomplete bundle branch block.

Initial treatment of these infants is first directed at decreasing pulmonary vascular resistance and preserving pulmonary blood flow. Prostaglandin E_1 should be initiated in an infant suspected of having Ebstein anomaly for maintenance of the patent ductus arteriosus.

Lesions Presenting as CHF

Truncus arteriosus

Patients with truncus arteriosus have only one great artery leaving the heart. This gives rise to the coronary arteries, aorta, and pulmonary arteries. There is a single semilunar valve, which is frequently regurgitant or stenotic. Patients with truncus arteriosus always have an associated large ventricular septal defect, and left and right ventricular pressures are equal. In addition, systemic and pulmonary arterial pressures are equal, resulting in pulmonary hypertension. Pulmonary arterial flow is frequently increased leading to pulmonary congestion and interstitial edema.

Physical examination findings in truncus arteriosus include tachypnea and diaphoresis, especially with feedings. As the pulmonary vascular resistance falls over the first few days of life, these symptoms become more prominent and patients frequently have a component of CHF as a result of the increased pulmonary blood flow. Mild cyanosis may be present. Pulses are bounding because of diastolic runoff into the pulmonary arteries. A right ventricular impulse is palpable at the left lower sternal border. Usually, a murmur and systolic ejection click is heard within the first several days of life because of the high-flow state.[6]

Chest radiography shows cardiomegaly and evidence of increased pulmonary blood flow, including pulmonary vascular congestion and interstitial edema. A right-sided aortic arch may be present. Truncus arteriosus should be strongly suspected in the setting of a right-sided aortic arch, a systolic ejection click, increased pulmonary vascular markings, and mild cyanosis.

Echocardiography is the modality of choice for diagnosis and reveals the large ventricular septal defect, single great artery, dysplastic truncal valve, and the divergence of the pulmonary arteries from the truncus. Doppler echocardiography can identify stenosis or regurgitation across the truncal valve. Initial stabilization of these patients involves treatment of CHF, as outlined previously.

Total anomalous pulmonary venous return

TAPVR occurs when the pulmonary veins do not connect to the left atrium and instead drain into other embryologic venous structures that would typically involute in the setting of correct pulmonary vein attachment to the left atrium. Anomalous pulmonary venous return is total or partial. Partial anomalous pulmonary venous return has some pulmonary veins draining normally to the left atrium and some "anomalous" pulmonary veins draining to other venous structures in the thorax. In patients with TAPVR, none of the pulmonary veins drain into the left atrium. The four forms of TAPVR are (1) supracardiac, (2) cardiac, (3) infracardiac, and (4) mixed. With all forms of TAPVR, an atrial septal defect is required for any blood to reach the left side of the heart. There is mixing of oxygenated and deoxygenated blood in the right atrium, and thus the blood that crosses the atrial septal defect to the left heart is not fully oxygenated. There is an increase volume load to the right atrium, which results in dilation of the right atrium, right ventricle, and pulmonary arteries.

Physical examination findings in neonates with TAPVR include mild to moderate cyanosis. As the pulmonary vascular resistance decreases after birth, signs of CHF develop with tachypnea and diaphoresis. Pulmonary rales and a hepatomegaly may be found. Patients with infradiaphragmatic TAPVR typically present more acutely than other subtypes and are more likely to become hemodynamically unstable.

Findings on chest radiograph include an enlarged cardiac size with increased pulmonary vascular markings. In cases of supracardiac TAPVR the cardiac silhouette resembles a figure eight or snowman in shape because of the dilated vertical vein and superior vena cava. As with other lesions, echocardiography is the standard diagnostic modality for diagnosing TAPVR and determining the location and drainage of all four pulmonary veins is essential.

Initial treatment of TAPVR should focus on management of heart failure. Some infants present with cyanosis as the chief complaint and may be started on prostaglandin E_1 as a stabilizing maneuver. TAPVR is the only cause of neonatal cyanosis that may be worsened by administration of prostaglandin E_1. In the presence of a prostaglandin E_1 infusion, pulmonary blood flow increases further through the patent ductus arteriosus causing worsening pulmonary vascular congestion and edema. If a cyanotic child with suspected congenital heart disease has worsening respiratory distress after initiation of prostaglandins, TAPVR should be suspected.

Ventricular septal defect

Ventricular septal defect, defined as a hole in the ventricular septum, is the most common congenital heart defect in children. At birth, the pressures in the right and left ventricles are equal, there is no shunting, and the ventricular septal defect may not be detected. As the pulmonary vascular resistance decreases after birth, blood begins to flow through the defect from the left ventricle to the right ventricle and recirculate through the lungs. As the shunt volume increases, both ventricles and the left atrium dilate, and right ventricular volume overload may cause hepatomegaly or pulmonary congestion. In the setting of a large defect, tachypnea and failure to thrive ensue. Pulmonary hypertension occurs when the high left ventricular pressure is transmitted through the defect to the pulmonary circulation.

History and physical examination components vary depending of the size, and resulting hemodynamic significance, of the defect. Patients with a small ventricular septal defect have a loud, holosystolic murmur, usually audible starting shortly after birth. They are generally otherwise asymptomatic. Patients with a moderate-to-large ventricular septal defect typically present with poor weight gain. They are often dyspneic and diaphoretic, especially with feedings. Feeding problems and irritability are common, and infants may be misdiagnosed with colic or gastroesophageal reflux. These infants also have hepatomegaly, and systemic perfusion can be compromised.[21]

Chest radiographs may demonstrate cardiomegaly and increased pulmonary blood flow as CHF develops. Echocardiography is the most accurate tool for diagnosing and characterizing a ventricular septal defect. An echocardiogram can also evaluate the hemodynamic significance of the lesion, including direction and volume of flow across the ventricular septum.[22]

Patent ductus arteriosus

In this abnormality, the ductus arteriosus remains persistently open after birth. Because the aortic pressure exceeds the pulmonary arterial pressure throughout the cardiac cycle, there is a continuous flow of blood from the aorta to the pulmonary artery. Postnatal increases in pulmonary blood flow in the setting of prematurity can lead to pulmonary edema, loss of lung compliance, and deterioration of respiratory function, which ultimately leads to chronic lung disease. Large amounts of left-to-right shunting through the ductus may also increase the risk of intraventricular hemorrhage, necrotizing enterocolitis, and death.[23] Persistent patent ductus arteriosus is much more common in premature infants and in patients with lung disease.[24] Genetic factors, environmental exposures, such as medications, and prenatal infections, such as rubella, may also play a role in persistent patency.[25]

Patients with symptomatic patent ductus arteriosus typically present as dyspneic, especially with activity. The hallmark physical finding in patients with a patent ductus arteriosus is a murmur, described as continuous and "machinery-like." Peripheral pulses are typically bounding. Some patients present primarily in atrial fibrillation because of chronic and progressive left atrial enlargement.

Chest radiographs in patients with patent ductus arteriosus can be normal or may display cardiomegaly with increased pulmonary vascular markings. Electrocardiogram is often normal in patients with small shunts but may show sinus tachycardia, atrial fibrillation, left ventricular hypertrophy, or left atrial enlargement with moderate-to-large shunts. Diagnosis can be made and the degree of shunting can be verified by echocardiography.

Stabilization of a symptomatic patient with a patent ductus arteriosus can generally be achieved with digoxin and diuretics. Afterload-reducing agents, such as angiotensin-converting enzyme inhibitors, may also improve clinical status. Patients presenting with arrhythmias, such as atrial fibrillation or flutter, should be treated with antiarrhythmics or cardioversion and maintained on antiarrhythmics, β-blocking medications, and anticoagulants as indicated.

Most patients have spontaneous closure of their ductus in the first days to months of life. However, if it does not close within the first year, it is very unlikely to do so spontaneously. At that point, intervention to promote closure is recommended to prevent long-term pulmonary complications and infective endocarditis, for which these patients are at increased risk. Nonselective cyclooxygenase inhibitors, such as indomethacin or ibuprofen, are generally used to induce ductus closure, but these may be less effective in severely premature infants.

Congenital Cardiac Arrhythmias

Supraventricular tachycardia

Supraventricular tachycardia is the most common symptomatic arrhythmia in the pediatric population, and 60% to 80% of these patients present in the first year of life.[8] The tachycardia is most commonly narrow complex, and the rate is typically greater than 220 beats per minute, but it can be up to 300 beats per minute. Atrioventricular reentrant tachycardia, including the Wolff-Parkinson-White syndrome, can result from an accessory bypass tract between the atria and ventricles. Atrioventricular nodal reentrant tachycardia occurs when there is a reentrant pathway within the atrioventricular node. Most patients with supraventricular tachycardia have structurally normal hearts, but 25% have an associated congenital heart defect. Presenting complaints with sustained tachycardia include irritability and feeding intolerance. If the duration of tachycardia is prolonged, the patient may develop CHF. Diagnosis is established by characteristic findings on electrocardiogram. A narrow-complex tachycardia with a rate of 220 to 300 beats per minute or regular sinus rhythm with a Wolff-Parkinson-White pattern, characterized by a short PR interval and a slurred, delta-shaped initial segment of the QRS complex, on electrocardiogram is highly suggestive of the diagnosis.

Initial treatment for supraventricular tachycardia includes attempts at blocking the atrioventricular node, because most of the supraventricular tachycardias involve the atrioventricular node as part of the electrical circuit. Vagal maneuvers can be attempted first, such as application of a bag of ice to the face. Adenosine, a potent atrioventricular nodal blocker, is the drug of choice for supraventricular tachycardia. It is successful at terminating supraventricular tachycardia in 80% to 90% of children. The initial dose is 0.1 mg/kg to a maximum of 6 mg and subsequent doses should be 0.2 mg/kg to a maximum of 12 mg. Other medication options include digoxin and procainamide. Verapamil should not be used in infants. An unstable child in supraventricular tachycardia should be rapidly direct-current cardioverted using 0.5 to 1 J/kg.

Stable children in sinus rhythm can be discharged home with pediatric cardiology follow-up. Patients may go home on an antiarrhythmic, such as digoxin or propranolol, but this decision should be made in consultation with pediatric cardiology. Many infants outgrow their supraventricular tachycardia by 1 year of age. Patients with persistent episodes of tachycardia after 1 year and despite aggressive medical therapy may require radiofrequency catheter ablation.

Long QT syndrome

Congenital long QT syndrome is a genetic disorder characterized by prolongation of the QT interval on electrocardiogram. This leads to a propensity for developing torsades de pointes polymorphic ventricular tachycardia in the setting of adrenergic stimulation. Long QT syndrome is highly genetically linked and is principally caused by mutations of the genes encoding potassium and sodium ion channels or proteins associated with these channels.

Patients with long QT syndrome often present primarily with palpitations, syncope, cardiac arrest, or sudden death. These patients are typically young and otherwise healthy. Any patient with palpitations, syncope, cardiac arrest, or sudden death requires that a thorough family history be obtained. In the setting of a family history of cardiac events at a young age or unexplained syncope or death, long QT syndrome needs to be strongly considered.

A 12-lead electrocardiogram should be obtained to confirm the diagnosis. QT interval should be measured, and an age- and gender-specific corrected QT interval (QTc) should be calculated. Patients with a QTc of greater than 500 milliseconds and symptomatic episodes are highly likely to have disease. A symptomatic patient with a borderline QTc of 440 to 500 milliseconds needs further evaluation.[26–28]

β-Blockers are the therapy of choice for long-term management of long QT syndrome to blunt the adrenergic surges associated with deterioration of sinus rhythm to torsades de pointes and then to ventricular fibrillation. Patients should be counseled to avoid activities associated with increased catecholamine release including exercise and swimming, high emotions, loud noise, or sudden awakening from sleep. In symptomatic patients with a QTc greater than 440 milliseconds, urgent referral to pediatric cardiology is imperative. Patients with a QTc greater than 500 milliseconds require cardiology consultation while still in the emergency department. In consultation with pediatric cardiology, these patients should be admitted to the hospital pending placement of the cardioverter-defibrillator or may possibly be discharged home with a portable external defibrillator and family education regarding its use. All first-degree relatives of definitively diagnosed patients should be screened for the disorder with electrocardiogram.[29]

Complete heart block

Congenital complete heart block in infants and children is relatively uncommon and in up to 30% patients there are associated structural heart defects.[8] Most of these patients are diagnosed en utero. Maternal risk factors include systemic lupus erythematosus. Acquired complete heart block is most typically a result of cardiac surgery for congenital heart disease; myocarditis; or infectious etiologies, such as Lyme disease.

Patients with symptomatic complete heart block present with signs and symptoms of hypoperfusion, including syncope or sudden death. Physical findings include bradycardia and cannon waves in the neck, generated by atrial contraction against closed tricuspid valves.

Diagnosis is achieved by electrocardiogram. Complete heart block as a result of Lyme carditis has a low morbidity, resolves spontaneously, and does not require any specific treatment. Definitive treatment for other causes of complete heart block is placement of a permanent pacemaker. In a hemodynamically unstable patient in the emergency department, sedation and transcutaneous pacing may be required.

SPECIAL CONSIDERATIONS IN THE TREATMENT OF ADULTS WITH CONGENITAL HEART DISEASE

As our surgical techniques, understanding of multisystem effects, and medical management of congenital heart disease have improved, the duration of survival with congenital heart disease has increased. The prevalence of severe congenital heart disease in adults increased 85% between 1985 and 2000, significantly outpacing the prevalence in the pediatric population.[30] Special circumstances, including pregnancy in a patient with congenital heart disease, must be considered as women with congenital heart disease live to childbearing age and beyond. In addition, adult patients with congenital heart disease may present to the emergency department with decompensation of their chronic cardiac conditions. Most of the acute presentations of adults with congenital heart disease involve heart failure, respiratory compromise, and dysrrhythmias.

Patients with long-standing congenital heart disease may develop CHF. Left-sided and right-sided lesions may be treated very differently in the setting of heart failure. Patients with primarily left-sided disease, including left ventricular dysfunction and aortic or mitral valve disease with ether low cardiac output or left atrial hypertension, may benefit substantially from positive pressure ventilation. Positive pressure increases intrathoracic pressure, decreasing afterload and allowing for more effective forward flow of blood. In contrast, patients with right-sided lesions likely decline further with the initiation of positive pressure ventilation. As intrathoracic pressure is increased, systemic vascular return to the heart decreases. This lowers cardiac preload and leads to decreased cardiac output and circulatory collapse. The remainder of supportive measures applicable to all other patients presenting with CHF including nitrates, diuretics, supplemental oxygen, and positive inotropy also apply to patients in heart failure with congenital heart disease.

Adult patients with congenital heart disease may develop pulmonary complications, such as pulmonary artery hypertension. Unrepaired systemic-to-pulmonary vascular connection, such as ventricular septal defect, patent ductus arteriosus, or atrioventricular canal, can result in increased pressure through the pulmonary vasculature. Known as Eisenmenger syndrome, these patients go on to develop cyanosis and its associated complications, such as polycythemia, headaches, blurred vision, and strokes. Shortness of breath ensues, and hemoptysis is not uncommon with advanced disease. Supplemental oxygen, digitalis, diuretics, phlebotomy, and anticoagulation may help mitigate some of the symptoms and complications of the disease. However, once the pathophysiologic changes have occurred, the process is generally progressive and irreversible.[31]

More than 50% of patients with congenital heart disease develop arrhythmias in their lifetime. Arrhythmias are the leading cause of hospital admissions for adults with congenital heart disease, and they constitute a significant predictor of mortality.[30] For patients with compromised cardiac output at baseline, loss of synchronous atrioventricular activity can cause hemodynamic compromise and collapse. Treatment is supportive, and intervention should be in collaboration with an electrophysiologist comfortable in the management of patients with congenital heart disease.

SUMMARY

Pediatric congenital heart disease comprises a wide spectrum of structural defects. These lesions, although many, tend to present in a limited number of ways. An infant presenting with profound shock, cyanosis, or evidence of CHF should raise the suspicion of congenital heart disease. Although most congenital lesions are diagnosed in utero, the emergency physician must be aware of these cardinal presentation because patients present in the postnatal period around the time that the ductus arteriosus closes. Aggressive management of cardiopulmonary instability combined with empiric use of prostaglandin E_1 and early pediatric cardiology consultation is essential for positive outcomes.

REFERENCES

1. Hoffman JI. Congenital heart disease: incidence and inheritance. Pediatr Clin North Am 1990;37(1):25–43.

2. Hoffman JI, Kaplan S. The incidence of congenital heart disease. J Am Coll Cardiol 2002;39(12):1890–900.

3. Pelech AN, Neish SR. Sudden death in congenital heart disease. Pediatr Clin North Am 2004;51(5):1257–71.

4. Sander TL, Klinkner DB, Tomita-Mitchell A, et al. Molecular and cellular basis of congenital heart disease. Pediatr Clin North Am 2006;53(5):989–1009.

5. Nora JJ. Etiologic aspects of heart diseases. In: Adams FH, Emmanouilides GC, Riemenschneider TA, editors, Moss' heart disease in infants, children, and adolescents, vol. 4. Baltimore (MD): Williams & Wilkins; 1989. p. 15–23.

6. Cooper JJ, Enderlein MA, Tarnoff H, et al. Asymmetric septal hypertrophy in infants of diabetic mothers: fetal echocardiography and the impact of maternal diabetic control. Am J Dis Child 1992;146:226–9.

7. Grifka RG. Cyanotic congenital heart disease with increased pulmonary blood flow. Pediatr Clin North Am 1999;46(2):405–25.

8. Burton DA, Cabalka AK. Cardiac evaluation of infants. The first year of life. Pediatr Clin North Am 1994;41(5):991–1015.

9. Reddy SC, Saxena A. Prostaglandin E1: first stage palliation in neonates with congenital cardiac defects. Indian J Pediatr 1998;65(2):211–6.

10. Barron DJ, Kilby MD, Davies B, et al. Hypoplastic left heart syndrome. Lancet 2009;374(9689):551–64.

11. Aboulhosn J, Child JS. Left ventricular outflow obstruction: subaortic stenosis, bicuspid aortic valve, supravalvar aortic stenosis, and coarctation of the aorta. Circulation 2006;114(22):2412–22.

12. Moss AJ. Clues in diagnosing congenital heart disease. West J Med 1992;156(4): 392–8.

13. Skinner J, Hornung T, Rumball E. Transposition of the great arteries: from fetus to adult. Heart 2008;94(9):1227–35.

14. Donnelly LF, Hurst DR, Strife JL, et al. Plain-film assessment of the neonate with D-transposition of the great vessels. Pediatr Radiol 1995;25:195–7.

15. Shinebourne EA, Babu-Narayan SV, Carvalho JS. Tetralogy of Fallot: from fetus to adult. Heart 2006;92(9):1353–9.

16. Apitz C, Webb GD, Redington AN. Tetralogy of Fallot. Lancet 2009;374(9699): 1462–71.

17. Strife JL, Sze RW. Radiographic evaluation of the neonate with congenital heart disease. Radiol Clin North Am 1999;37(6):1093–107.

18. Attenhofer Jost CH, Connolly HM, Dearani JA, et al. Ebstein's anomaly. Circulation 2007;115(2):277–85.

19. Paranon S, Acar P. Ebstein's anomaly of the tricuspid valve: from fetus to adult: congenital heart disease. Heart 2008;94(2):237–43.

20. Celermajer DS, Cullen S, Sullivan ID, et al. Outcome in neonates with Ebstein's anomaly. J Am Coll Cardiol 1992;19(5):1041–6.

21. Frommelt MA. Differential diagnosis and approach to a heart murmur in term infants. Pediatr Clin North Am 2004;51(4):1023–32.

22. Minette MS, Sahn DJ. Ventricular septal defects. Circulation 2006;114(20): 2190–7.

23. Hamrick SE, Hansmann G. Patent ductus arteriosus of the preterm infant. Pediatrics 2010;125(5):1020–30.

24. Bose CL, Laughon MM. Patent ductus arteriosus: lack of evidence for common treatments. Arch Dis Child Fetal Neonatal Ed 2007;92(6):F498–502.

25. Schneider DJ, Moore JW. Patent ductus arteriosus. Circulation 2006;114(17): 1873–82.

26. Zareba W, Cygankiewicz I. Long QT syndrome and short QT syndrome. Prog Cardiovasc Dis 2008;51(3):264–78.

27. Roden DM. Clinical practice. Long-QT syndrome. N Engl J Med 2008;358(2): 169–76.

28. Khan IA. Clinical and therapeutic aspects of congenital and acquired long QT syndrome. Am J Med 2002;112(1):58–66.

29. Moss AJ. Long QT syndrome. JAMA 2003;289(16):2041–4.

30. Allen CK. Intensive care of the adult patient with congenital heart disease. Prog Cardiovasc Dis 2011;53:274–80.

31. Rosenzweig EB. Eisenmenger's syndrome: current management. Prog Cardiovasc Dis 2002;45(2):129–38.

Index

Note: Page numbers of article titles are in **boldface** type.

A

Acute coronary syndrome(s), anticoagulant therapy in, 706, 707
    antiplatelet therapy in, 702
    ß-blockers in, 703
    cardiac biomarkers in, 690, 692–693
    cardiac ischemia in, 689
    clinical history screening in, 691–692
    clinical presentation and diagnostic approaches in emergency department, **689–697**
    continuum of, 690–691
    definitions of, 699–701
    electrocardiogram in, 692
    emergency department treatment of, **699–710**
    extent of testing in, 693–695
    follow-up percutaneous coronary intervention in, 705–706
    initial treatment of, 701–703
    morphine in, 703
    nitroglycerin in, 703
    non-ST-elevation myocardial infarction within, 690–691, 702
    non-ST-segment, percutaneous coronary intervention in, 706–708
        treatment of, 706–708
    patient screening for, 691–693, 694
    potential, physical examination in, 692
    primary, 699–700
    secondary, 700
    ST-elevation myocardial infarction within, 690–691, 700–701
        criteria for, 700
    supplemental oxygen in, 702
Airway management, in cardiac arrest recuscitation, 715
American Heart Association Guidelines 2010, 711–712
    evidence in support of, 712–715
Angiography, coronary CT, in "low-risk" chest pain, 725
Antiarrhythmics, in atrial fibrillation, 751–752
Anticoagulant therapy, in acute coronary syndromes, 706, 707
Anticoagulation, in atrial fibrillation, 753–754
Antiplatelet therapy, in acute coronary syndrome, 702
Aortic aneurysm, abdominal, causes and risk factors for, 794
        clinical presentation of, 795
        diagnostic modalities in, 795
        treatment of, 795–796
    thoracic, 797

Emerg Med Clin N Am 29 (2011) 829–835
doi:10.1016/S0733-8627(11)00104-0
0733-8627/11/$ – see front matter © 2011 Elsevier Inc. All rights reserved.

emed.theclinics.com

United States Postal Service

Statement of Ownership, Management, and Circulation
(All Periodicals Publications Except Requestor Publications)

1. Publication Title
Emergency Medicine Clinics of North America

2. Publication Number
0 0 0 - 7 1 1 4

3. Filing Date
9/16/11

4. Issue Frequency
Feb, May, Aug, Nov

5. Number of Issues Published Annually
4

6. Annual Subscription Price
$264.00

7. Complete Mailing Address of Known Office of Publication *(Not printer) (Street, city, county, state, and ZIP+4®)*
Elsevier Inc.
360 Park Avenue South
New York, NY 10010-1710

Contact Person
Amy S. Beacham

Telephone *(Include area code)*
215-239-3687

8. Complete Mailing Address of Headquarters or General Business Office of Publisher *(Not printer)*
Elsevier Inc., 360 Park Avenue South, New York, NY 10010-1710

9. Full Names and Complete Mailing Addresses of Publisher, Editor, and Managing Editor *(Do not leave blank)*

Publisher *(Name and complete mailing address)*
Kim Murphy, Elsevier, Inc., 1600 John F. Kennedy Blvd. Suite 1800, Philadelphia, PA 19103-2899

Editor *(Name and complete mailing address)*
Patrick Manley, Elsevier, Inc., 1600 John F. Kennedy Blvd. Suite 1800, Philadelphia, PA 19103-2899

Managing Editor *(Name and complete mailing address)*
Barton Dudlick, Elsevier, Inc., 1600 John F. Kennedy Blvd. Suite 1800, Philadelphia, PA 19103-2899

10. Owner *(Do not leave blank. If the publication is owned by a corporation, give the name and address of the corporation immediately followed by the names and addresses of all stockholders owning or holding 1 percent or more of the total amount of stock. If not owned by a corporation, give the names and addresses of the individual owners. If owned by a partnership or other unincorporated firm, give its name and address as well as those of each individual owner. If the publication is published by a nonprofit organization, give its name and address.)*

Full Name	Complete Mailing Address
Wholly owned subsidiary of	4520 East-West Highway
Reed/Elsevier, US holdings	Bethesda, MD 20814

11. Known Bondholders, Mortgagees, and Other Security Holders Owning or Holding 1 Percent or More of Total Amount of Bonds, Mortgages, or Other Securities. If none, check box ☐ None

Full Name	Complete Mailing Address
N/A	

12. Tax Status *(For completion by nonprofit organizations authorized to mail at nonprofit rates) (Check one)*
The purpose, function, and nonprofit status of this organization and the exempt status for federal income tax purposes:
☐ Has Not Changed During Preceding 12 Months
☐ Has Changed During Preceding 12 Months *(Publisher must submit explanation of change with this statement)*

PS Form **3526**, September 2007 (Page 1 of 3 (Instructions Page 3)) PSN 7530-01-000-9931 **PRIVACY NOTICE**: See our Privacy policy in www.usps.com

---

13. Publication Title
Emergency Medicine Clinics of North America

14. Issue Date for Circulation Data Below
August 2011

15. Extent and Nature of Circulation

		Average No. Copies Each Issue During Preceding 12 Months	No. Copies of Single Issue Published Nearest to Filing Date
a. Total Number of Copies *(Net press run)*		1494	1186
b. Paid Circulation (By Mail and Outside the Mail)	(1) Mailed Outside-County Paid Subscriptions Stated on PS Form 3541. *(Include paid distribution above nominal rate, advertiser's proof copies, and exchange copies)*	696	748
	(2) Mailed In-County Paid Subscriptions Stated on PS Form 3541 *(Include paid distribution above nominal rate, advertiser's proof copies, and exchange copies)*		
	(3) Paid Distribution Outside the Mails Including Sales Through Dealers and Carriers, Street Vendors, Counter Sales, and Other Paid Distribution Outside USPS®	177	215
	(4) Paid Distribution by Other Classes Mailed Through the USPS (e.g. First-Class Mail®)		
c. Total Paid Distribution *(Sum of 15b (1), (2), (3), and (4))*	▲	873	963
d. Free or Nominal Rate Distribution (By Mail and Outside the Mail)	(1) Free or Nominal Rate Outside-County Copies Included on PS Form 3541	70	65
	(2) Free or Nominal Rate In-County Copies Included on PS Form 3541		
	(3) Free or Nominal Rate Copies Mailed at Other Classes Through the USPS (e.g. First-Class Mail)		
	(4) Free or Nominal Rate Distribution Outside the Mail (Carriers or other means)		
e. Total Free or Nominal Rate Distribution *(Sum of 15d (1), (2), (3) and (4))*	▲	70	65
f. Total Distribution *(Sum of 15c and 15e)*	▲	943	1028
g. Copies not Distributed *(See instructions to publishers #4 (page #3))*	▲	551	158
h. Total *(Sum of 15f and g)*		1494	1186
i. Percent Paid *(15c divided by 15f times 100)*	▲	92.58%	93.68%

16. Publication of Statement of Ownership
☐ If the publication is a general publication, publication of this statement is required. Will be printed in the **November 2011** issue of this publication. ☐ Publication not required

17. Signature and Title of Editor, Publisher, Business Manager, or Owner
Amy S. Beacham — Senior Inventory Distribution Coordinator

Date
September 16, 2011

I certify that all information furnished on this form is true and complete. I understand that anyone who furnishes false or misleading information on this form or who omits material or information requested on the form may be subject to criminal sanctions (including fines and imprisonment) and/or civil sanctions (including civil penalties).

PS Form **3526**, September 2007 (Page 2 of 3)

EmergencyMed **Advance**

All the latest emergency medicine news and research you need, all in one place

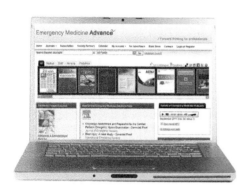

EmergencyMedAdvance.com is a new essential online resource offering valued high-quality content and news for the global community of Emergency Medicine professionals to save time and stay current—from physicians and nurses to EMTs.

Stay current
- Emergency Medicine news

Save time
- Access relevant articles in press from 16 participating journals

And more...
- Journals' profiles
- Personalized search results
- Emergency Medicine bookstore

- Upcoming meetings and events

- Search across 500+ health sciences journals
- Learn how to submit a manuscript

- Sign up for free e-Alerts
- Emergency Medicine jobs

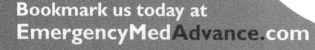

Printed and bound by CPI Group (UK) Ltd, Croydon, CR0 4YY

03/10/2024

01040457-0016